diabetes
EAT & ENJOY

The Authors

Christine Roberts is Director of Melbourne Dietetic Centre and Consultant Dietitian to hospitals, commercial organisations and in private practice. She has been involved with diet and diabetes for many years and has co-authored a number of papers. She was a member of the Working Party for Nutritional Resources, Diabetes Australia, in 1988. She co-authored the successful *Food for Sport Cookbook* and the *Healthy Heart Cookbook* (for the National Heart Foundation). She was also a contributor to Prof. Pincus Taft's book, *Diabetes Mellitus*.

Jennifer McDonald is consultant to a number of hospitals and other organisations. She has been involved in writing many publications for people with diabetes.

She has co-authored a number of scientific papers dealing with diet and diabetes, in association with other top researchers in the field. Her most recent, *Temporal Study of Metabolic Change when Non-Insulin Diabetes changed from low to high carbohydrate-fibre diet*, was published in the American Journal of Clinical Nutrition, 1988.

Margaret Cox has been involved in both research and clinical work with people with diabetes for many years. For three years she was nutrition co-ordinator at the Lions International Diabetes Institute, one of Australia's leading diabetes research and educational organisations, and was involved in the development of diabetes education programs and educational resources for people with diabetes.

She co-authored the *Healthy Heart Cookbook* for the National Heart Foundation.

Acknowledgements

There are a number of people who have helped and encouraged us in the writing of this book.

We would like first to acknowledge Diabetes Australia, their Health Care and Education Committee, and their National Marketing Committee, for their support.

We'd especially like to thank Jacqui Roberts for undertaking the difficult task of analysing the recipes and meal plans.

The expertise, advice and hard work of René Gordon, our original publisher, and her assistants Joy Bowers, Joslin Guest and Des Carroll have made this book a reality. The splendid colour photography is the work of Ann Creber, Lyn Zeeng and Lynda Patullo and we appreciate their skill and creativity.

Most importantly, we thank our families, and especially our husbands Noel Roberts, Michael Hall and Jack Cox – without their support, patience, encouragement and understanding, we could never have completed *Eat and Enjoy*.

Christine Roberts, Jennifer McDonald, Margaret Cox

diabetes
EAT & ENJOY

Christine Roberts • Jennifer McDonald • Margaret Cox

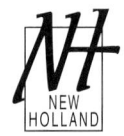

NEW HOLLAND

First published in Australia in 1990 by
New Holland Publishers Pty Ltd
Sydney • London • Cape Town • Singapore

Produced and published in Australia by
New Holland Publishers Pty Ltd
3/2 Aquatic Drive Frenchs Forest
NSW 2086 Australia

Copyright © 1990 Christine Roberts, Jennifer McDonald, Margaret Cox
Reprinted 1990, 1992 (twice)
Revised edition 1995
Reprinted 1996 (twice), 1998

Photography by Lyn Zeeng, Melbourne
Food styling Ann Creber, Melbourne
Layout and design Lynda Patullo, Green Poles Design, Melbourne
Typeset by DOCUPRO, Sydney
Printed in Singapore by Kyodo Printing Co. Pte Ltd.

National Library of Australia
Cataloguing in Publication Data

Roberts, Christine.
   Eat & enjoy: diabetes, what to eat and why: plus! more
   than 200 delicious recipes.

   New ed.
   Includes index.
   ISBN 1 86436 049 6.

   1. Diabetes – Diet therapy. 2. Diabetes – Diet therapy –
   Recipes. I. McDonald, Jennifer. II. Cox, Margaret.
   III. Title. IV. Title: Diabetes, what to eat and why.
   V. Title: Eat and enjoy.

616.4620654

All rights reserved. No part of this publication may be reproduced, stored in a retrieval system or transmitted, in any form or by any means, electronic, mechanical, recording or otherwise without the written permission of the copyright owners.

All meal plans in this book have been presented as samples only. Anyone wishing to follow these meal plans should first seek the advice of a qualified dietitian.

Cover photograph: J.B. Fairfax Press Pty Ltd/Ashley Mackevicius

TABLE OF CONTENTS

INTRODUCTION

KNOWLEDGE IS SWEET
What is diabetes?............................8
Types of diabetes..........................10

MANAGING DIABETES TODAY
The golden rules for diabetes.....................12
Understanding the principles
 of good nutrition 13
Guidelines to choosing food........................16

ON THE SHELVES
Artificial sweeteners......................25
'Diabetic' or 'carbohydrate modified'
 products..........................27
Low-kilojoule (low-calorie) products...........27
'Sugar-free' products......................28
Making sense of food labels 28
Better cereal choices 30

PLANNING YOUR MEALS
Sample meal plans.......................35
Timing your meals 39
Eating out 40
Treats and special occasions 41
Travel............................41
Shift work..........................41

SPECIAL NEEDS
Hypoglycaemia 42
What to do if you are ill............................44
High Blood Pressure......................45
High Blood Fat Levels 46
Pregnancy and diabetes......................47
Children and adolescents...........................47
Vegetarians with diabetes..........................49
Exercise, sport and diabetes......................51
How to modify recipes................................54

PLEASURES OF THE TABLE
Breakfasts.. 57
Appetizers and Snacks........................ 61
Soups... 70
Entrées and Light Meals....................... 79
Fish and Seafood 87
Meats and Poultry............................... 96
Meatless Dishes 120
Vegetable Side Dishes 131
Salads.. 146
Sauces, Dressings and Marinades 154
Desserts 167
Baking.. 188
After-Dinner treats 197
Drinks 199

The Detailed Food Value List 201

Eat & Enjoy

INTRODUCTION

As dietitians working with people with diabetes, we are constantly being asked to provide individuals with all the information they need about diet, cooking and eating. In the course of our work over the years, we were very aware how little simple, straightforward and up-to-date information there was about the relationship between food and diabetes.

Many people with diabetes don't have enough detailed, yet easily understood, information about the way in which the food they eat affects the control of diabetes, and this makes them unsure of how to plan or prepare their meals.

In the past few years, there have been major changes in the principles of eating for people with diabetes. Where in the past, people with diabetes were treated as being different, today we realise that the ideal diet for everyone is perfect for people with diabetes too.

Clearly there was a need for a book that explained simply the relationship between diabetes and food, laid out the guidelines needed for good management today, and included delicious and healthy recipes ideal for everyone, not just those with diabetes.

Eat & Enjoy does just that. Through this book we hope that you will have more confidence in your ability to maintain good health and enjoy the pleasures of the table.

Christine Roberts, Jennifer McDonald, Margaret Cox

SO WHO HAS DIABETES?

More and more people are being diagnosed with diabetes, so it is difficult to give accurate information about the number of people with diabetes in Australia. However, it is estimated that approximately 600,000 people have NIDDM (non-insulin dependent diabetes mellitus), and a further 105,000 have IDDM (insulin dependent diabetes mellitus).

WHERE TO GO FOR FURTHER HELP

DIETITIANS

- Your state branch of the Dietitians' Association of Australia.
- Look under 'Dietitian' in the Yellow Pages or other telephone directory.
- Ask your local doctor if he or she knows of a particular dietitian to refer you to.
- Contact your community health centre.
- Telephone your local hospital.
- Enquire at your State or Commonwealth Health Department.

DIABETES AUSTRALIA

DIABETES AUSTRALIA is the national co-ordinating organisation providing a unique partnership between consumers – the people with diabetes – research organisations, doctors and other health professionals with a special interest in diabetes.

Look under DIABETES AUSTRALIA in your telephone directory. DIABETES AUSTRALIA will provide information on the following:

- Member organisations and the services they provide
- Diabetes education programs
- Diabetes camps
- National Diabetic Supplies Scheme (subsidised syringes, needles and reagent test strips)
- National magazine *'Diabetes Conquest'*
- Additional membership advantages

KNOWLEDGE IS SWEET

Diabetes mellitus is not new. It may be as old as humanity. Certainly, it has been with us throughout recorded history, but only in 1921 did we learn to treat it with some effectiveness. And only in the past decade have we devised a new way of eating for people with diabetes. In the past 70 or so years, diabetes has changed from being a life-threatening condition to one that requires a change of lifestyle and, where necessary, medication.

WHAT IS DIABETES?

You need to know what diabetes is before you can take an active part in managing your own health care.

'Diabetes' comes from the ancient Greek word for 'siphon', referring to the large amount of sugar-containing urine passed by people with uncontrolled diabetes, and 'mellitus' for the characteristic sweet taste of the urine. **Diabetes (more accurately diabetes mellitus) is simply too much sugar in the blood.**

This sugar is in the form of **glucose**. Diabetes occurs when the system which controls the amount of glucose in the blood no longer works properly.

But where does it all begin? **Everyone** has glucose in their blood all the time. It provides energy (or fuel) to keep the body working, much like the petrol in a motor car.

Where does glucose come from?

Glucose comes from the food we eat. When we eat carbohydrate **(sugars and starches)**, our bodies convert it into glucose.

Some of the foods rich in carbohydrate:

- Breads, cereals and biscuits
- Pulses (such as dried peas, beans and lentils)
- Starchy vegetables (such as potatoes)
- Rice and pasta
- Fruit
- Milk
- Sugar
- Foods with sugar added, such as cakes, sweet biscuits, confectionery, sweetened soft drinks and canned fruit.

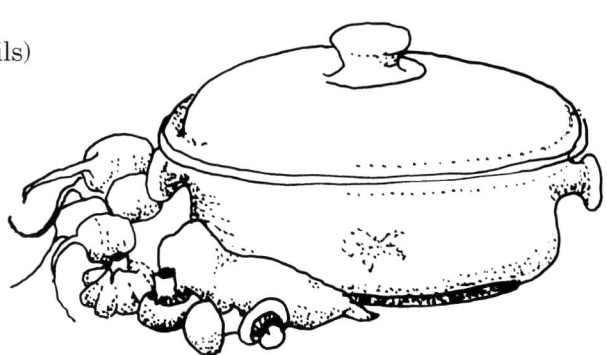

The digestive system breaks down carbohydrate to make glucose. The glucose is then absorbed into the bloodstream directly from the digestive tract or gut.

What happens to the glucose?

The blood carries the glucose to your body tissues (for instance, your brain, lungs, heart, liver, kidneys and muscles). There, the glucose passes from your blood into the tiny cells that make up body tissues, but the only way in which this can happen is with the help of the hormone insulin. On the wall of each tiny cell are special key holes or receptor sites. The insulin attaches itself to the glucose in the blood and locks itself into the receptor site in much the same way as you would use a key to open a door. This allows the glucose to pass through the cell wall into the cell where it is used for fuel.

Insulin is produced by the pancreas, a small gland that lies behind the stomach. Scattered throughout the pancreas are clusters of specialised cells, the Islets of Langerhans, which make and store insulin, and then release it into the bloodstream as needed. The pancreas, despite its small size, also produces digestive juices which help your body break down food as it passes through the gut.

After you have eaten, digested and absorbed food containing carbohydrate, the amount of glucose in your blood increases. In response to this, the pancreas releases the correct amount of insulin into your blood to carry the extra glucose into the cells. The amount of glucose in your blood then returns to its pre-meal level. At least, that's the way the system is supposed to work.

If you don't have diabetes, your blood glucose level never goes too high or too low, no matter how much or how little carbohydrate you eat. The system balances itself.

What happens when diabetes develops?

When the body produces little or no insulin, or the insulin it does produce is unable to carry glucose into your body cells, you develop diabetes.

With your normal glucose regulating system out of order, your level of blood glucose keeps on increasing. When it reaches a certain level, the body attempts to tackle the problem by passing the extra glucose out of your body via your urine. This is called 'glycosuria' — literally 'glucose urine'. Not surprisingly, with it can come symptoms such as:

- Passing large amounts of urine by day and night. This is called polyuria meaning 'much urine', and nocturia meaning 'night urine' as a way of getting rid of the excess sugar.
- Feeling very thirsty most of the time and having a dry mouth, the result of the large urine output.
- Drinking excessively (polydipsia) in response to thirst.
- Excessive tiredness due to the lack of available fuel to the cells.
- Losing weight because the normal fuel, glucose, is not available and the body breaks down fat stores.

- Itchiness and infections resulting from bacteria feeding on the extra glucose in blood and urine.
- Blurring of vision due to the effect of the high blood glucose on the fluid levels in the eye.

A medical examination will then reveal a high blood glucose level, in other words, a diagnosis of diabetes.

> *A high blood glucose level is known as hyperglycaemia, from 'hyper', meaning excessive and 'glycaemia' for sugar in the blood.*

What is a Normal Blood Glucose Level?

A normal blood glucose range for a person without diabetes is between 3.5 and 5.9 mmol/litre.

A fasting blood glucose level greater than 7.8 mmol/litre or a random (that is, not fasting), glucose level greater than 11.1 mmol/litre confirms a diagnosis of diabetes. (WHO recommendations)

NB: Fasting blood glucose is checked when you have been without food or drink for 10-12 hours. A random test can be taken at any time, regardless of whether you have eaten or not.

TYPES OF DIABETES

There are two main types of diabetes:

- Insulin-Dependent Diabetes Mellitus (IDDM) — Type 1
- Non-Insulin Dependent Diabetes Mellitus (NIDDM) — Type 2

Insulin-Dependent Diabetes Mellitus (IDDM) — Type 1

IDDM can develop at any age, but usually does so in childhood, during the teens or in early adulthood. What causes it is still unknown, but it may be caused by a virus which leads to the destruction of the Islets of Langerhans within the pancreas. Whatever the cause, the pancreas stops making insulin and symptoms usually appear quickly and severely.

If not treated promptly, your blood glucose level rises. As the glucose cannot get into the cells, your body begins burning up its fat stores too quickly (ketosis) and your breath smells of acetone. You may vomit, become dehydrated and feel drowsy. Left untreated, you will eventually lapse into a coma.

About 15 per cent of all people with diabetes have this type. The treatment is a combination of insulin injections and the healthy diet we present in this book. It is necessary to inject insulin, because if you were to take it by mouth it would be destroyed by your digestive juices long before it could be absorbed and used.

Non-Insulin Dependent Diabetes Mellitus (NIDDM) — Type 2

This is by far the more common of the two types of diabetes. It develops slowly and symptoms, if any, are likely to be less extreme than with IDDM. The only sign may be a high blood glucose level (hyperglycaemia) picked up on routine testing by your doctor.

NIDDM usually develops in people over the age of 40. It accounts for about 85 per cent of all cases. There is often a family history of diabetes.

A number of factors may influence the development of NIDDM, most importantly:

Family history, age, overweight, stress, alcohol abuse and inactivity.

With this type of diabetes, the pancreas makes some insulin, but not enough. Alternatively, excess body fat stops the insulin from carrying glucose into the body's cells.

Treatment for NIDDM is simply a healthy diet and exercise. If this is not enough to control the blood glucose then oral medication or insulin may be given. For the overweight person with this type of diabetes, **losing weight is the most important part of treatment**.

Even with well-controlled diabetes, insulin or extra oral medication may be needed during periods of illness, after surgery or emotional distress.

> *Diabetes tablets and how they work*
>
> *Diabetes tablets (oral hypoglycaemic agents) help lower your blood glucose level. They don't contain insulin, but help the body make more insulin or help you use the insulin you have more effectively.*

What happens if diabetes remains uncontrolled?

If your blood glucose level remains high or fluctuates excessively over a period, this may damage the blood vessels that supply your eyes, kidneys, heart and other organs and nerves, especially in your legs and feet. Learning how to manage your diabetes and to achieve good control is the best way to avoid these complications.

MANAGING DIABETES TODAY

Essentially good management of diabetes focuses on three major approaches:

- Diet
- Diet and diabetes tablets
- Diet and insulin injections
- Regular exercise makes an important difference to all people with diabetes and to your sense of well-being and general health.

Exactly which approach is most beneficial for you will depend on what type of diabetes you have, your weight, age and your blood glucose level.

There are two other important guidelines which will keep you fit and in good health:

- **Regular monitoring of your blood or urine glucose levels** helps you get to know your body and how it is coping with diabetes. It shows you the effect food, exercise and medication have on your blood glucose level (BGL), and helps you adjust them as necessary.
- **Regular visits to your doctor, dietitian and/or diabetes educator** — your partners in ongoing health care.

What can diet do for diabetes?

Food is important in keeping healthy, whether we have diabetes or not. However, most people don't pay enough attention to their basic nutritional needs. Diabetes highlights the importance of a well-balanced eating pattern.

If you have diabetes, there are three important benefits to be had from a nutritionally sound diet:

- Firstly, it helps you achieve and maintain good control of your blood glucose level.
- Secondly, it helps you regulate your body weight.
- Thirdly, it helps prevent or delay the onset of any of the long-term problems linked with diabetes.

THE GOLDEN RULES FOR DIABETES

The way to keep healthy now and in the future is to follow these Golden Rules:

- **Understand your diabetes and how to manage it.** Ask questions. Don't be shy or worry that you seem 'stupid' or are being a bother. No matter how 'silly' your question, ask it. And keep on asking until you are entirely satisfied that you understand your diabetes and know what to do to manage it. If, like so many people, you tend to go blank when seeing the dietitian, doctor or diabetes educator, sit down before your visit and write out all your questions and concerns. Take your list with you and go through it item by item.

These people are often busy and, if you need extra time, make an appointment for a less busy time. Alternatively, ask for a double appointment. Make sure you understand exactly what the prescribed treatment is supposed to do, and exactly how to follow it. You can also take a parent, friend or partner to help you remember what was said.

- **Keep your blood glucose level under control.** The best way of doing this is to eat sensibly, exercise regularly and take your medication correctly. Check your blood glucose levels regularly and have your doctor or diabetes educator do this at regular intervals.

- **If you are overweight, make losing weight a goal.** If you are slim, stay slim. There is no magic to losing weight. Basically, you need to make sure that you eat fewer kilojoules (calories) than your body burns up. You probably know whether you are eating too much, but if you are unsure of how to cut down on kilojoules (calories) without losing out on good nutrition, look at the meal plans in this book.

  Once you are slim, keep a careful watch on what you eat; it's all a matter of balance. You need to eat just enough to fuel your body through its normal daily routine, so concentrate on those things that provide your body with enough nutrients to keep it functioning perfectly. Remember, you can do this and still enjoy varied and tasty meals.

- **Be as physically active as possible**, keeping in mind your age, general health and your ability to exercise. This is not a call to becoming a super-athlete; simply by taking a brisk walk round the block twice a day you can keep fit. You may prefer to swim a few laps, play bowls or tennis, ride your bicycle or walk to the local shops instead of driving. But whatever exercise you choose, and whatever level of physical activity you find most comfortable, make it a regular part of your life. The benefits are immense.

UNDERSTANDING THE PRINCIPLES OF GOOD NUTRITION

Food is an important part of life — it is a necessity and it should be a pleasure. Diabetes need not change either of these aspects.

What we eat is a very individual matter. It's one of those areas where personal choice is allowed a wide expression. How you feel at any particular moment, your tastes, your cultural background and lifestyle all have an effect on your food choices.

The enjoyment we get from food should be matched by its value as a source of nourishment. It's the sort of thing we all are becoming more aware of, but may well ignore. However, when you develop diabetes, you have the opportunity to reappraise what you eat and improve your eating habits with immediate and significant benefits.

Foods provide a range of different textures, flavours, colours and nutritional value, and eating a variety will ensure the best combination for good health. The nutrients in food include protein, fat, carbohydrate, vitamins, minerals, fibre and water, all of which are essential for continued good health. It may be of help to know what these different nutrients do, and why they are vital.

PROTEIN

- Is an important part of all body tissues, enzymes, hormones and the immune system.
- You need protein for body growth and repair.
- Has only a small role as a body fuel.
- The richest sources are meat, poultry, fish, seafood, dairy products, eggs, nuts, seeds and pulses. You don't have to eat huge quantities of protein to meet your body needs.

FAT

- Provides fuel to keep the body working.
- Plays an important part in insulating and protecting the body's organs and other tissues.
- Transports other nutrients into and around the body.
- You need very small amounts daily to perform these important tasks. Major sources include butter, margarine, oils, meat, milk, cream and cheese.

CARBOHYDRATE

- Is the most important fuel source for all body tissues, especially the brain.
- Plays an important part in many body functions.
- Comes in two main forms — sugars and starches. Sugars are found naturally in fruit, milk and honey, and are added as sweeteners to many foods such as confectionery, cakes, soft drinks and jams. You find starches in breads, cereals, grains, vegetables and pulses.

VITAMINS

- Help the body produce fuel from carbohydrate, fat and protein.
- Work in combination with protein in growth and repair of body tissues.
- Play an essential part in body functions.

There are two types:

- Water-soluble vitamins, that is, all B vitamins and Vitamin C, which are found widely in foods including fruits, vegetables, cereals, milk and meat.
- Fat-soluble vitamins — A, D, E and K — which are found in animal fats such as butter, other dairy products, meat, vegetable oils and margarines, wholegrain products, nuts and seeds.

MINERALS

- Form a major part of bones, teeth and body fluids such as blood.
- Play an essential part in body functions such as heart beat, muscle contraction, and in nervous system and fluid balance.
- Occur widely in foods such as meat and fish, milk and cheese, fruits, vegetables and cereal products.

FIBRE

- Used to be called roughage and is the part of plant foods which is not broken down by the digestive juices.
- Has several tasks, including keeping the digestive tract in good shape. In other words, it keeps our bowels functioning regularly and easily.
- Also helps fill the stomach, satisfies our appetite and helps to limit over-eating.
- Delays the onset of hunger by slowing both digestion and the rate at which our body absorbs nutrients. In particular, from the point of view of a person with diabetes, it slows the rate of absorption of carbohydrate from the gut, thereby helping to control the blood glucose level.
- Is invaluable in your diet. Eat lots of it. Good sources of fibre include wholegrain breads and cereals, fruits, vegetables and pulses.

WATER

- Is an essential part of every body function. About two-thirds of the body is water.
- We lose between one and three litres of water every day through the lungs and in urine, faeces and sweat. The body can survive only for a few days without replacing this loss.
- Is the best drink for health. Don't wait until you're thirsty. Drink at least six to eight cups of fluid a day, and you will feel the benefit.

Food as a fuel source

Food is the energy source or fuel that keeps our bodies working. The energy supplied by any food is measured in kilojoules (or calories). Energy comes from three particular nutrients in our food. We have ranked them in order of importance: carbohydrate; then fat; lastly protein.

Alcohol provides concentrated energy, but it isn't usually considered a nutrient and certainly isn't essential.

GUIDELINES TO CHOOSING FOOD

A good guide for choosing a healthy diet is set out in the Australian Dietary Guidelines. Follow these guidelines and you will be on the way to managing your health and your diabetes. The first five are particularly important if you have diabetes:

- Eat plenty of bread and cereals (preferably wholegrain), pulses, vegetables and fruit.
- Limit your sugar intake.
- Limit your fat intake.
- Limit the amount of alcohol you drink.
- Control your weight.

But don't ignore the rest. Here they are:

- Choose a nutritious diet from a variety of foods.
- Cut back on salt.
- Encourage breast feeding.
- Drink plenty of water.

And for women, teenage girls, athletes and vegetarians be sure to have enough iron and calcium to meet your additional needs.

In this section, we will explain why these guidelines are important to you.

EAT PLENTY OF BREADS AND CEREALS (ESPECIALLY WHOLEGRAIN), PULSES, FRUIT AND VEGETABLES

These foods offer a number of benefits, and should make up the bulk of your diet. They contain plenty of carbohydrate and fibre, vitamins and minerals and, if you eat them regularly, they will actually help control your diabetes. They will also help you control your weight because they are satisfying and bulky.

Important: Try to include at least three or four serves of high-carbohydrate, high-fibre food (as shown next) in every meal. If you are young and/or active, your carbohyrate requirements will be much higher. You may find that you need more carbohydrate at meals and/or high carbohydrate snacks to ensure you have enough carbohydrate in your body all through the day.

Rather than using accurately weighed or measured foods we have used average serves as a basis for carbohydrate intake. Experience has shown that as long you are **consistent** this can give you good control and make life easier.

We have used 1 slice of bread as a standard but you can increase your serves according to your individual needs. **Remember plenty of carbohydrate is the aim.**

CEREALS

Include bread, biscuits, breakfast cereals, rice, wheat, barley, oats, buckwheat, rye, pasta (such as spaghetti and noodles).

1 serve	= 1 slice of bread	= 4–6 dry biscuits
	= ¾ cup of cereal	= ½ cup of cooked pasta
	= ½ cup of cooked rice	

PULSES

Include dried beans (such as red kidney beans, borlotti, white, black-eyed, lima, haricot, cannellini, baked beans and soy beans), peas (such as split peas and chick peas) and lentils.

1 serve = ½ cup, cooked

VEGETABLES

Starchy vegetables include potatoes, sweet potatoes, sweetcorn and yams.

1 serve = ½ cup, cooked
= 1 medium potato

Vegetables, other than the starchy ones listed above, are low in carbohydrate, but high in fibre, and are a particularly rich source of minerals and vitamins. You should include plenty of them in your daily diet together with starchy vegetables.

FRUIT

Include all varieties.

1 serve = 1 large piece of fresh fruit
= ¾–1 cup stewed fruit

Some fruits are lower in carbohydrate than others. The list on page 202 will prove a useful guide.

All about Carbohydrate and Fibre-rich Food

Knowing about carbohydrate is important for you if you have diabetes. After all, carbohydrate breaks down into glucose, and balancing your blood glucose level is a vital part of your management.

It is useful for you to understand the difference between refined (simple) sugars such as sugar itself, and complex (unrefined) carbohydrate, such as in cereals, breads and pulses.

Refined sugars are low in nutrients while providing energy, whereas complex carbohydrate-rich foods provide many essential nutrients and fibre as well as energy. They should form the basis of your eating plan.

Serves of different carbohydrate foods have different effects on the blood glucose levels, even when they provide the same amount of carbohydrate, with some causing a quicker and higher rise in blood glucose levels than others.

Foods are rated according to the effect they have on blood glucose levels. This is known as the **glycaemic index.** Foods which cause a small rise in blood glucose levels have a low glycaemic index number. Foods which cause a greater rise have a higher glycaemic index number.

The best foods are those which have a low glycaemic index number, provided they are also low in fat.

Many factors affect the glycaemic index such as cooking, the amount of fat, the type of starch and fibre and the amount of processing.

What effect do these factors have?

Cooking - the more a food is cooked the easier it is for the body to break down the food and to absorb the carbohydrate and therefore the quicker the rise in blood glucose level.

Fat - foods high in fats often have a low glycaemic index. This is due to the fat slowing down digestion. **However, high fat intake is not recommended for people with diabetes.**

Starches - different starches are broken down and absorbed at different rates.

Fibre - helps slow down the digestion and absorption of starches.

Processing - the more a food is processed the easier it is for the body to break down the food and absorb the carbohydrate.

The foods that offer the most benefits to people with diabetes in terms of glycaemic index include:

- pulses, all varieties
- oat, barley and bran cereals
- breads containing large amounts of wholegrains such as pumpernickel, wholegrain rye and wheat
- barley, buckwheat, bulgar
- basmati rice and doongara rice (an Australian long grain variety)
- all pasta including spaghetti and noodles
- some fresh fruits such as apples, cherries, grapefruit, oranges, peaches, pears, plums and firm bananas
- some vegetables such as sweet potato, yam and sweetcorn.

It is recommended that at least one serve of food of low glycaemic index (as listed above) be included at each meal or one meal containing several foods of low glycaemic index be included daily. This helps to even out swings in blood glucose levels and leads to better control.

This information is current, but research continues and there may be further changes.

Fibre

As mentioned earlier, fibre is important in helping control your blood glucose level and regulating bowel function. To maximise your fibre intake:

- Choose wholegrain/wholemeal breakfast cereals. For the best choices see the list on page 201.

- Replace white rice and pastas with brown rice and wholemeal pastas. You'll be delighted with how tasty they are.

- Use more pulses in your cooking. Add them to soups, casseroles, salads, savoury dishes and dips.

- Make sure you eat vegetables every day (including the starchy ones). Use them in salads, soups, meat dishes and so on.

- Include at least two to three pieces of fruit in your daily eating plan. Preferably eat them fresh rather than cooked, and don't drink more than one **small** glass of fruit juice per day, as this is low in fibre.

- Leave vegetables and fruit unpeeled where possible, for maximum fibre.

LIMIT YOUR SUGAR INTAKE

An enormous number of the processed foods we eat contain added sugars. You will find sugar in many forms, some obvious, some less so, in many of the foods you buy such as cereals, biscuits, canned fruit, soft drinks, confectionary and chocolates. Sugars are high in kilojoules (calories) but often are low in other nutrients. This means that they can add to your weight without providing any useful nourishment.

Diabetes does not mean a total ban on sugars. You can eat small amounts as part of meals without making your blood glucose level rise excessively. In practice, this means that a scrape of jam on wholemeal toast or a little sugar used in your wholemeal cake recipe will do no harm.

You can also train your palate to prefer far less sugar than we have become accustomed to in our western diet.

Hints to help you cut down on sugars

- Always check product labels. Read the section *Making Sense of Food Labels* (page 28).

- Avoid sugar in tea, coffee or other beverages.

- Buy solid pack unsweetened canned fruit, fruit packed in water, or artificially sweetened canned fruit instead of fruit canned in natural juices or syrups.

- Water is the best thirst quencher. But if you must, use low-joule (low-calorie) soft drinks, flavoured mineral waters and cordials instead of the regular varieties.

Eat & Enjoy   *Introduction*

- If you want flavoured jellies, use the low-joule (low-calorie) products.
- If you like jam, marmalade or honey on your toast or bread, have some, but limit it to a scrape and forget the butter or margarine.
- In your cooking, look for recipes with very little or no sugar, fructose or honey. Our recipes will give you a guide to just how little sugar or sweetness you need to make food delicious. Remember, too, that fruit is a good source of sweetness. In many of our recipes you will see that we use fruit and fruit juices in recipes which traditionally are made with sugar.
- Low-fat fruit yoghurts are often surprisingly high in sugar. Choose those that are artificially sweetened or make your own by combining low-fat natural yoghurt and your choice of fresh or stewed fruits.
- There are many excellent artificial sweeteners on the market. These may be used to replace sugar.

LIMIT YOUR FAT INTAKE

Fat is a taste-enhancer, and we have become used to eating far too much of it. Not only do we use it knowingly by frying foods or by ladling on the cream; we also eat a great deal of fat unknowingly in processed foods. It is sobering to realise that a 100 gram (3 ounce) packet of potato crisps contains 40% fat and 2385 kJ (570 cal) and that a plain unsweetened shop-bought biscuit may have as much as 20% fat and 262 kJ (63 cal).

Because fat is the most concentrated form of energy we eat, there is a danger that a diet high in fats will add unnecessary kilojoules (calories). It may lead to weight gain.

Heart and circulation problems are often associated with a diet high in fats. Reduce your fat intake, and this may reduce your chances of developing such problems.

Remember that eating too much fat may have a direct effect on insulin activity in your body, causing an increase in your blood glucose level.

Just as you don't have to give up sweetness in your foods, you don't have to give up fats altogether. **It is important, however, that you limit your intake.** Cutting back begins in the kitchen, and continues at the table.

Hints to help you use less fat

- Select lean cuts of meat and remove skin and fatty deposits from poultry.
- Use the absolute minimum oil or fat in cooking. If possible, don't use any added fat at all.
- When you must use fat, use a brush to spread a thin layer of fat onto your pan, or use a cooking spray.
- Grill or roast meat on a rack to allow the fat to drip away.
- For soups and casseroles, drop meat into boiling water to seal it rather than browning it in fat or oil.

- Spread butter or margarine very thinly on bread and biscuits, or leave it off. Use ricotta, cottage cheese, a little avocado or a scrape of low-fat cream cheese as a spread instead.

- Use low fat dairy products in preference to the regular varieties.

- Use 'no-oil', 'low-oil' or 'low-joule' (low-calorie) salad dressings instead of oily ones or mayonnaise. Better still, use lemon juice or vinegar with herbs to add zest to your salads. Turn to our *Dressings* section (page 160) for ideas.

- Learn to use fresh or dried herbs and spices to add flavour to food instead of butter or oil.

- Avoid adding oil or fat to vegetables during or after preparation. For instance, when you mash potato or other vegetables, don't add butter, margarine or cream. Use low-fat milk. Wrap your vegetables in foil with herbs, or try dry baking them in the oven in their own skins.

- If you like sour cream as a vegetable dressing, use low-fat leben or cottage cheese or low-fat natural yoghurt instead.

- Use our recipe for Creamy Whipped Topping (see page 165) instead of cream on desserts.

Our recipes reflect our recommendations; we use fat, where necessary, but sparingly. The recipes will convince you that you can eat wonderful, nutritious food and still cut down on fat.

Protein foods

Protein foods often contain fat, so be aware of this when you make choices. Consider the following:

MEAT, POULTRY, FISH

Protein is important to a healthy eating plan and you should include some every day. Many people eat far too much. You only need one or two small serves of protein daily.

By a small serve, we mean about 100 g (3 oz) of cooked meat or fish. To give you some idea of what this means, 100 g (3 oz) of steak is a piece about the size of an average hamburger pattie. If in doubt, at first weigh your meats or fish, or ask your butcher or fishmonger to weigh them for you.

When choosing protein foods, select those which are lower in fat, such as:

- **Lean** beef, veal, pork or lamb
- Chicken or turkey **without skin**
- Fish and seafood
- **Lean** game meat such as rabbit, buffalo, venison and kangaroo

To be classified as lean, meat should have minimal visible fat marbled through it, and you should trim off any fat around the meat **before** you cook it.

EGGS

Eggs are a good source of protein. They are low in fat, although the yolk is rich in cholesterol. Unless you have a high cholesterol level, you can eat three or four eggs a week. Two eggs make a good serve.

PULSES

Pulses are excellent as a source of protein and have the added advantage of being low in fat. They make an ideal alternative or addition to meat dishes. They are rich in carbohydrate and fibre, so include them often. Three-quarters of a cup of cooked pulses is a good serve size.

NUTS AND SEEDS

Nuts and seeds — and products made from them, such as peanut butter and tahine — are a valuable source of protein, but are high in fat, so eat them in small amounts.

MILK AND MILK PRODUCTS

Regular milk and dairy products are high in fat, but there are many low-fat products available and you would do well to use them:

- Skim or low-fat milks
- Skim or low-fat yoghurts, natural or artificially sweetened
- Skim or low-fat cheeses
- Low-fat ice creams.

When choosing low-fat cheeses, preferably choose those with less than 20 per cent fat. When choosing low-fat ice creams choose those with less than 4 per cent fat. Also try to avoid eating cream and sour cream — save them for special occasions and, even then, use them in small amounts.

Milk as a carbohydrate source

Milk and yoghurt contain the carbohydrate lactose (milk sugar). One cup of milk or yoghurt will give you roughly the same amount of carbohydrate as a slice of bread. The use of small amounts of milk such as that taken in tea or coffee need not be considered as a carbohydrate source, but a cup of milk or yoghurt makes a good alternative to other carbohydrate foods.

A Special Note on Milk

Dairy products are important sources of protein and calcium. Women, particularly, should be aware of the value of dairy products in helping protect them from osteoporosis (loss of calcium from bones). Calcium, of course, plays a vital part in good bone health.

Adult men should include 1½ cups of milk — 300 mL (½ pint) — or the equivalent in dairy products in their daily diet.

Children, adolescents, and adult women (including those who are pregnant, breast-feeding or post-menopausal) should double this. They should include at least three cups — 600 mL (1 pint) — of milk or the equivalent in dairy products in their daily diet.

*The following each contain **about** the **same quantity** of calcium:*

250 mL (8 fl oz) milk   200 mL (7 fl oz) yoghurt   40 g (1⅓ oz) piece of cheese

LIMIT THE AMOUNT OF ALCOHOL YOU DRINK

Alcoholic drinks are high in kilojoules (calories), and can contribute to weight gain. They can also react with diabetes tablets or insulin, causing a drop in your blood glucose level. Too much alcohol taken regularly can lead to a rise in the fat level in your blood which increases risk of heart disease.

Having diabetes does not mean that you cannot drink alcohol at all. It simply means moderation and good sense. **If you drink alcohol, then we recommend that you do not drink more than one or two standard alcoholic drinks a day.** By a 'standard' drink we mean a small — 200 mL (7 fl oz) glass of beer, a 140 mL (5 fl oz) glass of wine, a 30 mL (1 fl oz) nip of spirits such as whisky, vodka or gin or a 60 mL (2 fl oz) glass of dry vermouth or dry sherry.

Remember that many drinks such as beer, sweet wines and liqueurs also contain significant amounts of carbohydrate which may increase your blood glucose level. So, it's best to choose a dry rather than a sweet wine, and to drink low-alcohol beer rather than the regular ones.

Don't be lulled into a false sense of security by drinking 'diabetic' or 'diet beers'. These contain a large amount of alcohol and kilojoules (calories) and should be treated as if they were ordinary alcoholic drinks when it comes to quantity.

Here are some preferred choices in alcoholic drinks:

Dry wines (riesling, chablis, burgundy, claret, graves); brut champagnes; spirits; low-alcohol beers (2.5 per cent or less); dry fortified wines, such as dry vermouth and dry sherry.

A note about mixers:

When using mixers, be aware that all the regular soft drinks contain a large amount of refined sugar, and we do not advise their use. But water and low-joule (low-calorie) mixers can be used freely, as follows:

- *Water*
- *Soda water*
- *Unflavoured mineral water*
- *Low-joule (low-calorie) drinks including tonic, dry ginger ale, bitter lemon, cola-flavoured drinks and lemonade.*

Most importantly, don't drink alcohol on an empty stomach. **Always** eat some starchy food when you drink, for example, dry biscuits with your whisky, a meal with your wine.

Unsweetened fruit juice and milk contain carbohydrate and are useful as mixers in situations where no better source of carbohydrate is available, such as a slice of bread or a dry biscuit.

If you are taking diabetes medication, and you drink alcohol without having carbohydrate, your blood glucose level may drop too low, leading to **hypoglycaemia or 'hypo' which can be serious and require urgent action**. On page 42 we tell you more about hypoglycaemia, how to prevent and treat it. You will also find more information on alcohol on page 204.

CONTROL YOUR WEIGHT

Being overweight makes diabetes more difficult to control. The extra body fat alters the cell receptor sites as described on page 9 so that they are unable to accept the combination of insulin and glucose. As a result, blood glucose levels remain too high.

Fortunately, once you lose excess weight, the receptor sites are reactivated, allowing insulin to be taken up effectively so that your blood glucose level can be controlled without medication or with minimal amounts of tablets or injected insulin.

If you are overweight, losing weight is the key to good diabetes control, and should be a priority. It will also benefit your overall health. Check the following chart to see whether you need to maintain or lose weight.

TABLE OF ACCEPTABLE WEIGHTS-FOR-HEIGHTS 2.5 cm = 1 in 1 kg = 2.2 lb [14 lb = 1 stone]

Height cm	Weight kg	Height cm	Weight kg	Height cm	Weight kg
140	39–49	158	50–62	176	62–77
142	40–50	160	51–64	178	63–79
144	41–52	162	52–66	180	65–81
146	53–53	164	54–67	182	66–83
148	44–55	166	55–69	184	68–85
150	45–56	168	56–71	186	69–86
152	46–58	170	58–72	188	71–88
154	47–59	172	59–74	190	72–90
156	48–61	174	61–76		

Height (cm) without shoes   Body weight (kg) – in light clothing without shoes

Whether you need to maintain or lose weight, the guidelines given in this book will help you achieve your goal. If you need to lose weight you will have to reduce your kilojoule (calorie) intake.

By limiting your fat and sugar intake, and having more foods high in carbohydrate and fibre, you should be able to control your weight and still eat enough to satisfy your appetite.

While you are losing weight, it is important to maintain your health by eating regular meals that supply all your nutritional needs. Avoid crash diets and quick solutions — they offer no long term benefits. Developing a healthy eating pattern over a period will help you to achieve and maintain a lower weight.

Remember, in your quest for better health:
- *Eat regular meals each day.*
- *Include plenty of wholegrain bread, cereals, pulses, vegetables and fruit every day.*
- *Cut down on fats, concentrated sugars and alcohol.*
- *Reduce your weight if you are overweight; if you are slim, keep it that way.*
- *Eating should be a pleasure; make sure your meals have plenty of flavour and texture.*

Foreground: Ginger Pears, next Mixed Berry Salad with Lemon Cream, and Lemon Delicious above. Mocha Mousse served in the tall glass.

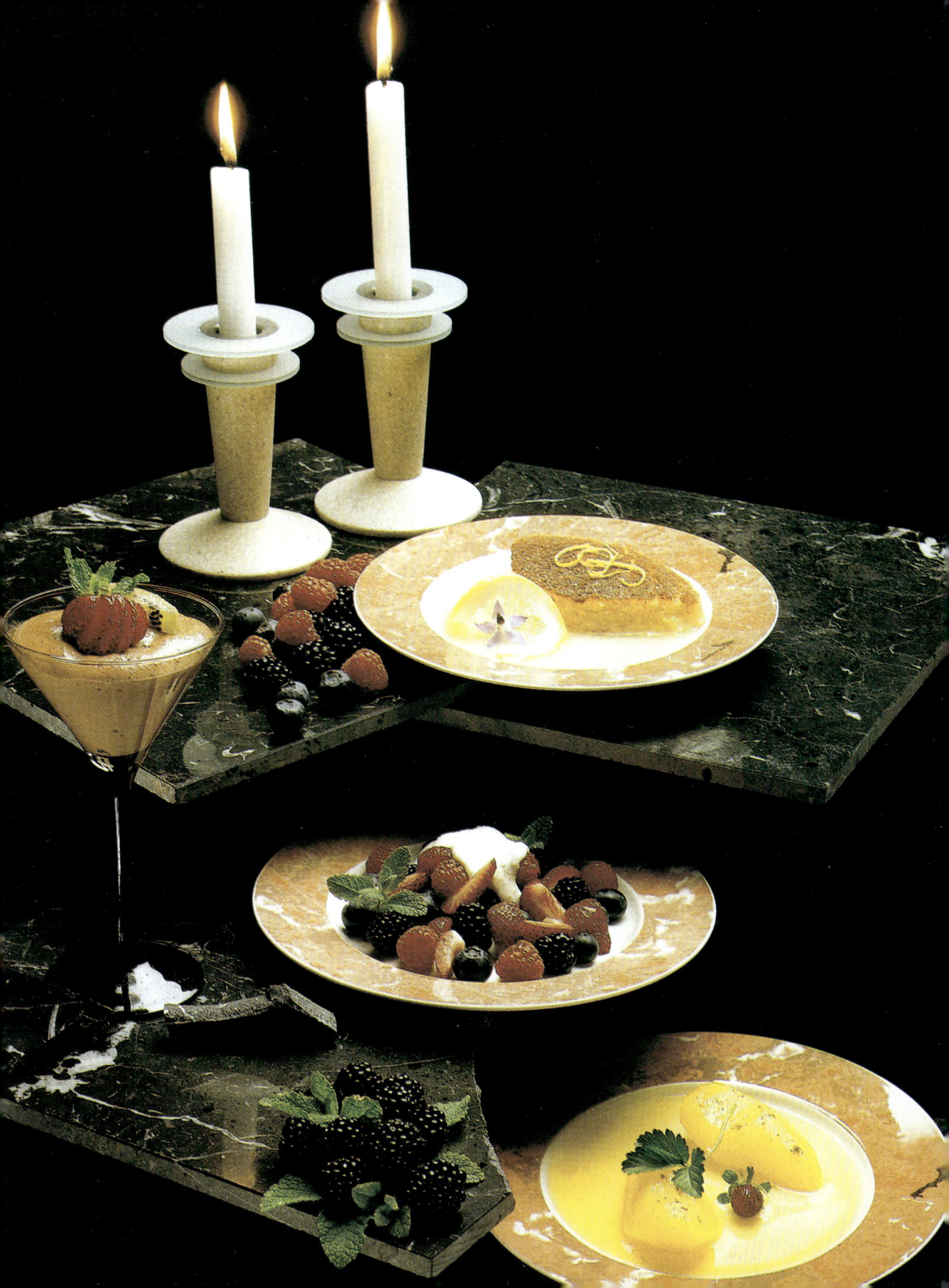

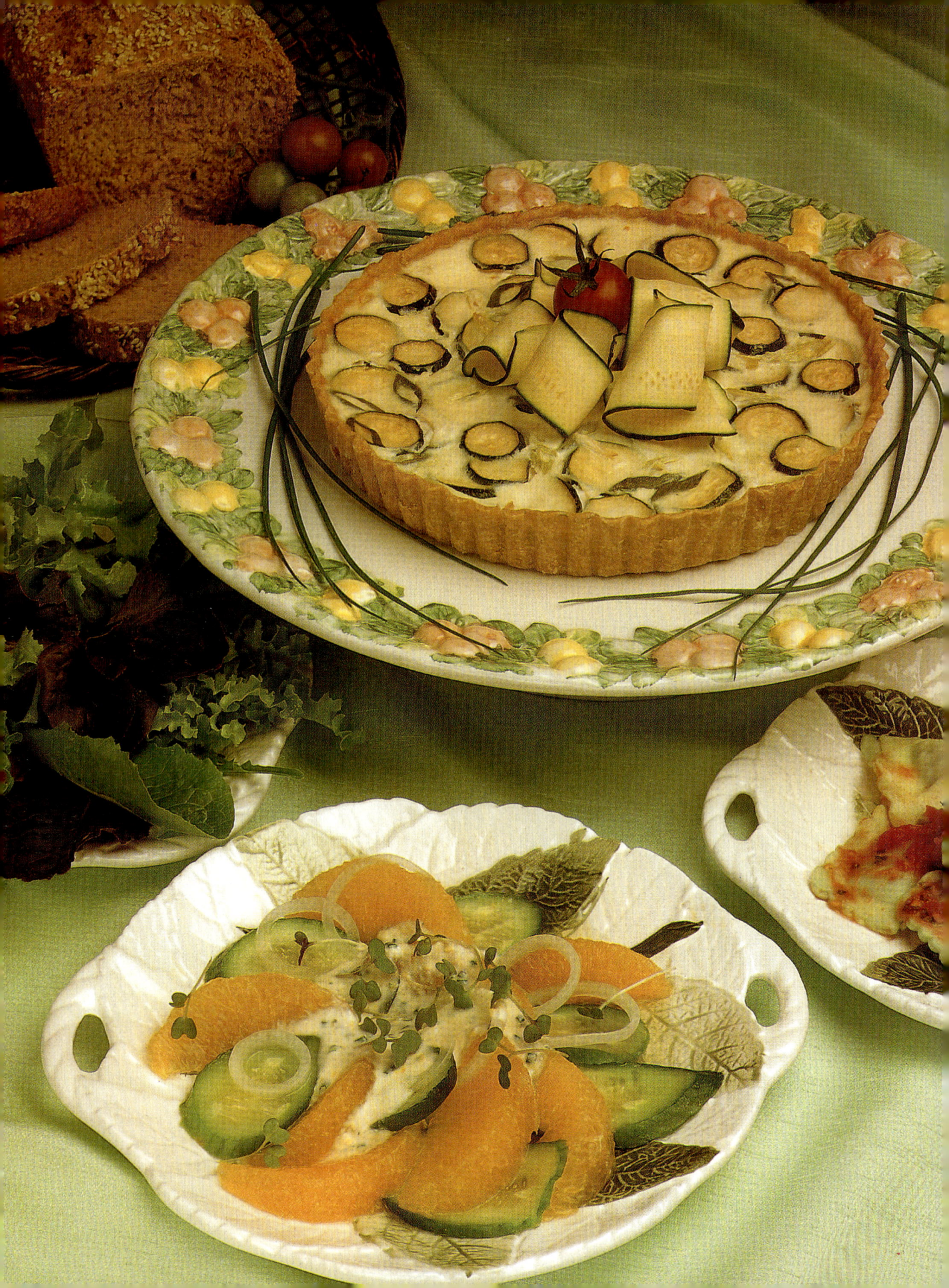

ON THE SHELVES

ARTIFICIAL SWEETENERS

Wherever possible, enjoy the natural sweetness of food. But if you must have added sweetness, you can use the many alternatives to sugar available on the market.

There has been some controversy about the safety of some of these products with prolonged and frequent use. However, these concerns have not been proved and overweight is considered a far greater risk to good health than any of these sweeteners.

Some artificial sweeteners contain kilojoules (calories) and others do not, or have very small amounts.

Artificial sweeteners which have negligible kilojoules (calories) include:

ACESULFAME - K (Trade name Sunett). 200 times sweeter than sugar, and has been available for the past 10 - 15 years.

It is used in a variety of manufactured food products such as fruit drinks and soft drinks, and in sweetened dairy products such as yoghurts. It is not available as a table sweetener.

It is not metabolised by the body, therefore does not contribute to energy intake.

Some people find it leaves a bitter after-taste as do saccharin and cyclamate.

ASPARTAME. It was discovered by chance when a scientist was researching ulcer drugs. For domestic use it is marketed as 'Equal' and we have used it in many of our recipes. Under the trade name 'Nutrasweet' it sweetens a host of commercially prepared foods and beverages.

Because it tends to break down under high heat or during lengthy cooking, aspartame is not suitable for cooking, unless you add it at the end of the process. This is not always possible, for instance in baking, and so other sweeteners should be used.

Aspartame is 180 times sweeter than sugar, dissolves in liquid (making it useful as a sweetener in tea and coffee), and has no unpleasant after-taste.

CYCLAMATE. This also was a chance discovery. In 1937 a scientist tasted sweetness on his cigarette after he had put it down accidentally on some white powder. When he checked, he discovered the sweetener, cyclamate.

Cyclamate is 30 times sweeter than sugar. It enjoyed considerable popularity for many years, but then became the focus of safety issues. In 1969 it was banned in the United States of America and the United Kingdom when it was implicated in possible liver and kidney damage in laboratory animals. However, the Carcinogen Assessment Group in the United States determined that cyclamate does not cause cancer in humans. Pending further research into other possible side effects, cyclamate remains banned in the United States although it is widely available in the rest of the world, including Australia.

Foreground: Orange and Cucumber Salad, to the right Spinach Ravioli with Fresh Tomato Sauce, in the centre a spectacular Crab and Zucchini Quiche, with sliced Quick Wholemeal Bread.

Cyclamate is soluble and therefore useful as a sweetener in hot and cold drinks. It does not have as strong an after-taste as saccharin, and does not lose its sweetening qualities when cooked.

SACCHARIN. The oldest of the artificial sweeteners, it was discovered in 1879 and went into commercial use in the early 1900s. It is 300 times sweeter than sugar; however, up to one in four people notice a bitter or metallic after-taste in foods sweetened with it. By mixing saccharin with cyclamate the taste can be improved. Saccharin is soluble and therefore useful as a sweetener; however, it is best added as late as possible in the cooking process to limit the development of any bitter after-taste.

In terms of safety, saccharin has been intensively studied and it would appear that, in the quantities any human is likely to take, it has no dangerous side effects.

SUCRALOSE. This new artificial sweetener has just been approved in Australia. It is 600 times as sweet as sucrose. Sucralose is made from sugar which has undergone a chemical process in which chlorine is added. Sucralose is not digested by the body and therefore does not have any effect on blood glucose levels or add any energy to the diet. The brand name for Sucralose is 'Splenda'.

Splenda™ is a powder that is a combination of sucralose and maltodextrin. Maltodextrin will cause a rise in blood glucose levels but is used in such small amounts in Splenda™ that it is suitable for people with diabetes. 1 teaspoon of Splenda™ contains only 8 kilojoules (2 calories). Splenda™ is stable to heat so it can be used in baked goods and has no bitter after-taste.

Artificial sweeteners supplying kilojoules (calories) include:

SORBITOL. It is manufactured commercially from glucose obtained from natural sources such as fruits. It is absorbed slowly into the bloodstream and, therefore, does not cause a major increase in blood glucose level, although it supplies as many kilojoules (calories) as other sugars. Because of the kilojoules (calories) it contains, we would recommend that you avoid or limit its use. Be aware, too, that more than 40 g (1½ oz) of sorbitol taken in a single day may have a laxative effect.

MANNITOL. This is a sugar alcohol made from mannose which is found in seaweed and some other natural products. It is approximately half as sweet as sugar and may have a mild laxative effect if you take more than 15 g (½ oz) a day. It contributes only about 8 kilojoules (2 calories) per gram because it is poorly absorbed.

FRUCTOSE. Occurring naturally in fruits and honey, it can be purchased as a white powder which is slightly sweeter than sugar, but contains the same amount of energy per weight.

Fructose is absorbed more slowly than sugar, so it does not increase the level of blood glucose as quickly or to the same extent following absorption. It also does not require as much insulin for its use in the body. For these reasons it is sometimes used to sweeten foods for people with diabetes; however, because of its energy content, and its overall effect on the blood glucose level, we recommend it be used sparingly and, preferably, not at all.

LACTOSE. Lactose or milk sugar is frequently used as a bulking agent to produce powdered artificial sweeteners which resemble sugar in appearance. It contributes the same amount of kilojoules (calories) as any other sugars. Use this type of sweetener with caution.

Read the labels of your sweeteners carefully. Many are made from combinations of sweeteners, or are bulked up with agents such as lactose.

TIPS AND TRAPS WHEN USING ARTIFICIAL SWEETENERS

- Artificial sweeteners are much sweeter than sugar, so you only need a small amount.
- Some people's taste buds are very sensitive to these products, and they describe a lingering bitter or metallic after-taste. Using a different sweetener or using less of the product may help you overcome this.
- Cyclamate and saccharin develop a bitter taste when boiled, particularly when cooked with fruit. Always add these sweeteners after the fruit has been cooked and has cooled. Where food is not boiled, for example, when baking an egg custard, the sweetener can be added before cooking.
- Aspartame loses its sweetness when heated and is not suitable for dishes which require heating.
- Aspartame loses its sweetness with prolonged storage in liquids. For example, soft drink sweetened with aspartame does not store well.
- Some sweeteners are mixed with other sugars such as lactose and glucose to reduce the concentration of their sweetness, and to enable you to sprinkle them. This adds kilojoules (calories), so use them sparingly.
- Some products are advertised as sugar free, but if you read the label, you will see that they contain quite large amounts of sweeteners such as sorbitol and fructose.

'DIABETIC' or 'CARBOHYDRATE MODIFIED' PRODUCTS

You will find many foods targeted at people with diabetes.

These fall into two main groups:

High fat - diabetic (carbohydrate modified) chocolates, ice creams and biscuits.

Low fat - jams, chutneys, pickles and sauces.

Generally, you will find that these specialised products are more expensive and do not taste as good as the regular variety.

Small amounts of either the regular or specialised alternatives are acceptable; **however those who are overweight should limit their use of the high fat group to an occasional treat.**

LOW-JOULE (LOW-CALORIE) PRODUCTS

These products are marketed for people who want to lose weight. They are suitable for people with diabetes and you can use them freely. Here are some of them:

- Low-joule (low-calorie) jams and jelly, low-joule (low-calorie) soft drinks and cordials, low-oil or no-oil salad dressings.

Eat & Enjoy   Introduction

'SUGAR FREE' PRODUCTS

Foods labelled as 'sugar free' are only free of added sugar, and they should not be confused with low-joule (low-calorie) products. Some are high in naturally occurring sugars such as fructose, lactose, grape juice, apple concentrate and pear juice. The kilojoule (calorie) value of these products can be as high as regular sweetened products; you should use them sparingly.

If you are still uncertain whether a product is suitable, read the label carefully and, if it appears high in these sugars, ask your dietitian for advice (see the next section for information on understanding labels).

MAKING SENSE OF FOOD LABELS

Many commercial foods which you can buy at the supermarket contain a lot of sugar and/or fat and may be low in fibre, making them unsuitable for you. But how do you know which ones they are?

Reading labels provides valuable information, but is not always as straightforward as it looks. You need to know how to interpret the information so you can make wise choices.

Ingredient list

There are food labelling laws in Australia which state that all ingredients in a product must appear on the label, listed in order of quantity. This means the ingredient used in the greatest amount is listed first, and that used in the smallest amount is listed last.

For example, let us look at a product label including the following ingredients: **Wheat flour, oats, beef fat, malt extract, sultanas, flavouring, salt.**

There is more wheat flour in this product than anything else, and less salt.

To help you decide which products are suitable or unsuitable, we have listed some of the names used for fat, sugar and fibre:

FAT	**SUGAR**		**FIBRE**
beef fat	apple concentrate	mannitol	bran
beef tallow	brown sugar	molasses	oatbran
butter fat	corn syrup	pear concentrate	ricebran
coconut cream	dextrose	sorbitol	rolled oats
coconut oil	glucose	sucrose	wheatgerm
copha	fructose	treacle	wheatmeal
corn oil	golden syrup	xylitol	wholegrain
cottonseed oil	grape concentrate		wholemeal
lard	honey		
margarine	invert sugar		
oil	lactose		
shortening	malt		
soya bean oil	malt extract		
vegetable oil	maltose		

28   Introduction   Eat & Enjoy

Nutrition information

Some products will also include a chart showing nutrient composition. This information is of greater value than the ingredient list as it is more accurate and allows you to make product comparison more easily.

The information given 'per 100 g' is easier to compare than the 'per serve' column.

Here are some examples of labels:

Example One

NUTRITION INFORMATION
Servings per package: 24. Serving size: 30 g (2 biscuits)

	Per Serving	Per 100g	2 BISCUITS WITH 1/2 CUP (125 ml) WHOLE MILK	SO GOOD
ENERGY (kJ)	410	1380	750	735
PROTEIN (g)	3.7	12.4	7.8	7.9
FAT (g)	0.8	2.7	5.5	5
CARBOHYDRATE				
TOTAL (g)	19.3	64.3	25	25.2
SUGARS (g)	0.7	2.3	6.4	2.7
SODIUM (mg)	80	270	153	149
POTASSIUM (mg)	105	350	297	280

in accordance with the regulations set out in the Australian Food Standards Code, the following information refers to the quantity of 60 g (4 biscuits) alone, and with 1 cup (250 ml) of whole milk or So Good Non-Dairy Drink.

60 g OF SANITARIUM WEET-BIX CONTAINS   * D. A. = Daily Allowance

	ALONE		WITH 1 CUP (250 ml) WHOLE MILK		SO GOOD	
	By weight (mg)	% D. A. *	By Weight (mg)	% D. A. *	By weight (mg)	% D. A. *
THIAMINE	0.55	50	0.65	59	0.66	60
RIBOFLAVIN	0.8	50	1.22	76	1.22	76
NIACIN	5.5	50	5.75	52	6.63	60
IRON	5.0	50	5.25	52	6.25	62

WeetBix Hi-Bran ingredients: Whole wheat, raw sugar, salt, malt extract, vitamins (niacin, thiamine, riboflavin), mineral (iron). No artificial flavouring or colourings.

At first glance you might think this product is unsuitable because sugar appears as the second ingredient. On closer inspection you can see that the sugar level fits well within the guidelines for a recommended cereal (see page 30).

Example Two

Baked beans in tomato sauce vegetarian ingredients: Navy beans, tomato puree, sugar, thickener (modified cornflour), salt, food acid (260), spices, water added.

NUTRITION INFORMATION

			PER SERVE 125 g	PER 100 g
Serving per package	6.0	Energy	480 kJ	384 kJ
Serving size	125 g	Protein	6.1 g	4.9 g
		Fat	0.9 g	0.7 g
		Carbohydrates – Total	21.5 g	17.2 g
		– Sugars	5.5 g	4.4 g
		Dietary Fibre	6.3 g	5.0 g
		Sodium	479 mg	383 mg
		Potassium	350 mg	280 mg

INGREDIENTS: NAVY BEANS 50%, TOMATO PUREE, SUGAR, THICKENER (MODIFIED MAIZE STARCH), SALT, SPICES, FOOD ACID (296), NATURAL COLOURS (150, 160e) WATER ADDED
SPC LIMITED, ANDREW FAIRLY AVE., SHEPPARTON, VICTORIA, 3630, AUSTRALIA

In this product, too, sugar appears fairly high on the list of ingredients, but on checking the nutrition information you can see that the amount of sugar per serve is quite low. Baked beans are also high in fibre and low in fat, making them an ideal food for people with diabetes.

Eat & Enjoy   *Introduction*

BETTER CEREAL CHOICES

Start your day right with cereal for breakfast. With the great number of products available, it is difficult to know which ones to choose. Your best choices are high in fibre and low in added sugar.

To help you make a sensible choice, we have listed those we recommend. This may not be a complete list as new products are coming onto the market all the time. For cereals not on the following list, read the labels and use our guidelines.

To be included on our **recommended** list, 100 grams (3 ounces) of cereal had to contain no more than 15 grams of sugar and at least 7.5 grams or more of dietary fibre.

Recommended

Unsweetened untoasted (natural) muesli

Kellogg's
- *All-Bran
- Balance Flakes
- *Bran Flakes
- *Mini-Wheats Whole Wheat
- Puffed Wheat
- *Ready Wheats
- *Sultana Bran
- *Sustain
- Wholegrain Wheatflakes

Sanitarium
- *Bran Bix
- Good Start
- Granola
- Granose
- Lite-Bix

Puffed Wheat
Weet-Bix
Weet-Bix High Bran
*Weet-Bix plus Oat Bran
Wheat Flakes
Wheat Germ

Uncle Toby's
- *Crunchy Oat Bran
- Fruit 'n Nut Weeties
- *High Fibre Oats
- *Instant Porridge Plus
- Oatflakes
- Organic Vitabrits
- *Raw Oat Bran
- *Shredded Wheat
- *Traditional Oats
- Weeties

* Gives a guide to some cereals with a low glycaemic index.

PLANNING YOUR MEALS

We've given you the guidelines, now comes the application. What you choose and the quantity you eat will depend on your energy requirements and your weight, as well as on that very important factor, your preferences.

YOUR ENERGY NEEDS

The following chart shows approximate energy needs for people of different age, sex and healthy weight.

If you are active your needs may be greater; if you are physically inactive your needs may be less.

Subject	Age years	Body mass kg (lb)	Energy kJ (cal)
Boys	11–15	41 (90)	12200 (2920)
	15–18	61 (134)	12600 (3000)
Girls	11–15	42 (92)	10400 (2500)
	15–18	55 (121)	9200 (2200)
Men	18–35		11600 (2775)
	35–55	70 (154)	10400 (2500)
	55–75		8800 (2100)
Women	18–35		8400 (2000)
	35–55	58 (128)	7600 (1820)
	55–75		6400 (1530)
Pregnant	18–35	+ 10 (22)	9000 (2150)
(Last 6 months of pregnancy)			

If you need further information or guidance discuss this with your dietitian.

YOUR CARBOHYDRATE, FAT AND PROTEIN NEEDS

The average Australian gets 35 per cent of his or her energy from **carbohydrate**. A healthier percentage is 50–60 per cent.

The average intake of energy from **protein** is 20–30 per cent and should be reduced to **15–20 per cent,** while the **fat** average of 45–55 per cent energy should be reduced to **30–35 per cent**.

The following chart gives you the amount of carbohydrate, protein and fat you need to eat to meet the recommended percentage intake for varying energy levels.

YOUR CARBOHYDRATE, PROTEIN AND FAT READY RECKONER

Energy (kJ)	(cal)	Carbohydrate 50–60% (g)	Protein 15–20% (g)	Fat 30% (g)
5000	1200	150–165	45–60	40
5650	1350	170–185	50–68	45
6300	1500	190–205	56–75	50
6900	1650	205–230	61–83	55
7550	1800	225–250	67–90	60
8200	1950	245–270	72–98	65
8800	2100	260–290	78–105	70
9400	2250	280–310	83–113	78
10,000	2400	300–330	89–120	80

MORE ABOUT CARBOHYDRATE

If you are already managing your diet, you may be doing it by various methods such as simply avoiding too much sugar and fat, or by measuring 'serves' of food which contain 10 g or 15 g of carbohydrate ('portions' or 'exchanges'). **The size of serves does not matter provided that you follow the principles of high carbohydrate and fibre, low fat and added sugar.**

The figures for carbohydrate that you are using may differ from the ones we give, but ours reflect the latest information. If your carbohydrate level is currently low and you increase it, you **may** find that your blood glucose levels are higher for a short while. Your medication may need adjusting temporarily. Discuss this with your doctor, educator or dietitian.

For good control of your blood glucose level, **older, inactive people** should eat **at least three or four serves of high-carbohydrate, high-fibre foods** at each of their three daily meals (45-60 grams of carbohydrate per meal).

Younger and/or **more active people** may need to eat five, six or more carbohydrate serves at each meal (at least 75 grams of carbohydrate per meal).

Remember that the high-carbohydrate, high-fibre foods include bread, cereals, pulses, vegetables and fruits. On pages 16–17 we have shown you approximate serve sizes. Each of the carbohydrate serves shown will give you approximately 15 grams of carbohydrate.

We have also detailed the carbohydrate content of each recipe in this book so you know how much carbohydrate you are eating at each meal. For instance, one serve of Bombay Burgers (recipe, page 81) will give you about 20 grams of carbohydrate. When you accompany this with a wholemeal roll, a green salad and a serve of fruit, you have an ideal meal containing 3–4 serves (about 60 grams) of carbohydrate. The addition of a bowl of Beef and Bean Soup (recipe, page 77) will increase this to five serves (about 75 grams) of carbohydrate.

Of course, your carbohydrate intake can be made up of half serves or double serves, depending on what suits you. Remember, the figures are only approximate, and you don't have to be precise.

Generally, we do not recommend snacking between meals for older, less active people. If you are young, active or involved in vigorous exercise, or if your medications make it necessary, you may need to include high-carbohydrate snacks in your eating plan. But remember, snacking can contribute unnecessary kilojoules (calories) which, in turn, can lead to putting on weight.

Below we have a simple meal plan which shows you how to put into practice the information we give. The carbohydrate-rich foods have been highlighted for easy identification. The quantities of food will vary from person to person, and your weight is the best guide.

Breakfast

1 serve **wholegrain cereal** with low-fat milk

1 serve **fruit**

1-2 slices **wholemeal toast** or **rye bread** with a scrape of margarine and a topping of your choice

Lunch

2 slices **wholemeal** or **rye bread** or **bread roll** with a scrape of margarine

1 thin slice of lean red meat or chicken (no skin) or tuna or salmon or egg or low-fat cheese

plenty of salad vegetables

1-2 serves **fruit**

Dinner

1 small serve lean red or white meat or fish

2 serves **starchy vegetables** or **rice** or **pasta**

plenty of non-starchy vegetables

1 serve **fruit** and or low-fat yoghurt

Bedtime snack

1 serve **wholemeal** or **rye bread** or **wholemeal biscuit**, and a scrape of margarine

and/or 1 cup low-fat milk as drink

This menu is, of course, rather plain, but it does show how to distribute your carbohydrate evenly through the day.

MEAL PLANS

You know your kilojoule (calorie) requirements, and how much of each of the nutrients you need daily. You also know that you should spread your carbohydrate through the day. The following pages show you how to take this information and convert it into food.

We have also given lists of foods which will give you information about food values and help you add variety and interest to your meals. You will find these on pages 201 to 204.

SAMPLE MEAL PLANS

Water, tea, coffee or other low-joule beverage may be drunk with or between meals as desired.

5000 kJ (1200 cal)

Breakfast
- 1 serve Meg's Muesli topped with 1 sliced banana and 100 mL low-fat milk
- 1 slice wholegrain bread spread with 1 tsp margarine and topped with sliced fresh tomato and black pepper

Lunch
- 1 sandwich made with 2 slices pumpernickel bread spread with 2 rounded tsp peanut butter and filled with chopped celery and lettuce
- 1 apple
- 2 mandarines

Dinner
- 1 serve Meatballs in Tomato Sauce accompanied by ½ cup cooked rice
- 1 serve Vegetables Julienne
- 1 serve Mocha Mousse

Nutritional Data
Energy & Nutrients: 5168 kJ 1234 cal, 154 g carbohydrate, 74 g protein, 38 g fat
Energy Ratio: 48% carbohydrate, 24% protein, 27% fat
Carbohydrate distribution: 47 g breakfast, 46 g lunch, 50 g dinner, 12 g from extra milk in beverages.

6300 kJ (1500 cal)

Breakfast
- 1 serve Meg's Muesli topped with 1 sliced banana and 100 mL low-fat milk
- 1 slice wholegrain bread spread with 1 tsp margarine and topped with sliced fresh tomato and black pepper
- 1 slice wholemeal toast spread with 1 tsp margarine and Date and Fig Spread

Lunch
- 1 sandwich made with 2 slices pumpernickel bread spread with 2 rounded tsp peanut butter and filled with chopped celery and lettuce
- 1 slice wholemeal bread spread with 1 tsp margarine and Vegemite
- 1 apple
- 2 mandarines

Dinner
- Orange Borscht Soup
- 1 serve Meatballs in Tomato Sauce accompanied by ½ cup cooked rice
- 1 serve Vegetables Julienne
- 1 serve Mocha Mousse

Nutritional Data
Energy & Nutrients: 6368 kJ 1521 cal, 194 g carbohydrate, 84 g protein, 48 g fat
Energy Ratio: 49% carbohydrate, 23% protein, 28% fat
Carbohydrate distribution: 63 g breakfast, 57 g lunch, 63 g dinner, 12 g from extra milk in beverages.

SAMPLE MEAL PLANS

Water, tea, coffee or other low-joule beverage may be drunk with or between meals as desired.

7550 kJ (1800 cal)

Breakfast
- 1 serve Meg's Muesli topped with 1 sliced banana and 100 mL low-fat milk
- 100 g low-fat fruit yoghurt
- 1 slice wholegrain bread spread with 1 tsp margarine and topped with sliced fresh tomato and black pepper
- 1 slice wholemeal toast spread with 1 tsp margarine and Date and Fig Spread

Lunch
- 1 sandwich made with 2 slices wholegrain bread spread with 2 rounded tsp peanut butter and filled with chopped celery and lettuce
- 1 sandwich made with 2 slices pumpernickel bread, one spread with 1 tsp margarine, the second with Creamy Yoghurt Dressing and filled with grated carrot and a sprinkling of sultanas
- 1 apple
- 2 mandarines

Dinner
- Orange Borscht Soup
- 1 serve Meatballs in Tomato Sauce accompanied by ½ cup cooked rice
- 1 serve Vegetable Julienne
- 1 serve Mocha Mousse

Bedtime Snack
- 1 slice wholegrain bread spread with 1 tsp margarine and Vegemite

Nutritional Data
Energy & Nutrients: 7527 kJ 1798 cal, 238 g carbohydrate, 95 g protein, 56 g fat
Energy Ratio: 51% carbohydrate, 22% protein, 28% fat
Carbohydrate distribution: 79 g breakfast, 74 g lunch, 63 g dinner, 12 g bedtime snack, 12 g from extra milk in beverages.

10000 kJ (2400 cal)

Breakfast
- 1 serve Meg's Muesli topped with 1 sliced banana and 100 mL low-fat milk
- 100 g low-fat fruit yoghurt
- 2 slices wholegrain bread, one spread with 1 tsp margarine and topped with fresh tomato and black pepper; the other with 1 tsp margarine and Date and Fig Spread

Morning Tea
- 1 serve wholemeal biscuits spread with 1 tsp margarine

Lunch
- 1 sandwich made with 2 slices pumpernickel bread each spread with 1 tsp margarine and filled with 2 rounded tsp peanut butter; chopped celery and lettuce
- 1 sandwich made with 2 slices wholegrain bread each spread with 1 tsp margarine and filled with grated carrot, a sprinkling of sultanas and Creamy Yoghurt Dressing
- 1 apple
- 2 mandarines

Afternoon Tea
- 2 peaches

Dinner
- Orange Borscht Soup
- 1 wholegrain roll (without margarine)
- 1 serve Meatballs in Tomato Sauce
- 1 cup cooked rice
- 1 serve Vegetables Julienne
- 1 serve Mocha Mousse
- 1 cup canned apricots (no added sugar)

Bedtime Snack
- 2 slices wholegrain bread each spread with 1 tsp margarine and Vegemite

Nutritional Data
Energy & Nutrients: 1006 kJ 2403 cal, 333 g carbohydrate, 114 g protein, 73 g fat
Energy Ratio: 54% carbohydrate, 19% protein, 27% fat
Carbohydrate distribution: 79 g breakfast, 13 g morning tea, 73 g lunch, 14 g afternoon tea, 119 g dinner, 23 g bedtime snack, 12 g from extra milk in beverages.

SAMPLE VEGETARIAN MEAL PLANS

Water, tea, coffee or other low-joule beverage may be drunk with or between meals as desired.

5000 kJ (1200 cal)

Breakfast
- 1 serve Meg's Muesli topped with 1 sliced banana and 100 mL low-fat milk
- 1 slice wholegrain bread spread with 1 tsp margarine and topped with sliced fresh tomato and black pepper

Lunch
- 1 sandwich made with 2 slices pumpernickel bread spread with 2 rounded tsp peanut butter and filled with chopped celery and lettuce
- 1 apple
- 1 mandarine

Dinner
- 1 serve Jumping Bean Bake
- 1 serve Tossed Salad
- 1 serve Mocha Mousse

Nutritional Data
Energy & Nutrients: 5076 kJ, 1213 cal, 160 g carbohydrate, 68 g protein, 35 g fat
Energy Ratio: 51% carbohydrate, 23% protein, 26% fat
Carbohydrate distribution: 47 g breakfast, 41 g lunch, 61 g dinner, 12 g from extra milk in beverages.

6300 kJ (1500 cal)

Breakfast
- 1 serve Meg's Muesli topped with 1 sliced banana and 100 mL low-fat milk
- 1 sliced wholegrain bread spread with 1 tsp margarine and topped with sliced fresh tomato and black pepper
- 1 slice wholegrain toast spread with 1 tsp margarine and Date and Fig Spread

Lunch
- 1 sandwich made with 2 slices pumpernickel bread spread with 2 rounded tsp peanut butter and filled with chopped celery and lettuce
- 1 slice wholegrain bread spread with 1 tsp margarine and Vegemite
- 1 apple
- 1 mandarine

Dinner
- Orange Borscht (prepared with vegetable stock rather than chicken)
- 1 serve Jumping Bean Bake
- 1 serve Tossed Salad
- 1 serve Mocha Mousse

Nutritional Data
Energy & Nutrients: 6283 kJ, 1501 cal, 201 g carbohydrate, 78 g protein, 45 g fat
Energy Ratio: 52% carbohydrate, 21% protein, 27% fat
Carbohydrate distribution: 63 g breakfast, 52 g lunch, 74 g dinner, 12 g from extra milk in beverages.

SAMPLE VEGETARIAN MEAL PLANS

Water, tea, coffee or other low-joule beverage may be drunk with or between meals as desired.

7550 kJ (1800 cal)

Breakfast
- 1 serve Meg's Muesli topped with 1 sliced banana and 100 mL low-fat milk
- 100 g low-fat fruit yoghurt
- 1 slice wholegrain bread spread with 1 tsp margarine and topped with sliced fresh tomato and black pepper
- 1 slice wholegrain toast spread with 1 tsp margarine and Date and Fig Spread

Lunch
- 1 sandwich made with 2 slices pumpernickel bread spread with 2 rounded tsp peanut butter and filled with chopped celery and lettuce
- 1 sandwich made with 2 slices wholegrain bread each spread with 1 tsp margarine and filled with grated carrot, a sprinkling of sultanas and Creamy Yoghurt Dressing
- 1 apple

Dinner
- Orange Borscht (prepared with vegetable stock rather than chicken)
- 1 serve Jumping Bean Bake
- 1 serve Tossed Salad
- 1 serve Mocha Mousse

Bedtime Snack
- 1 slice wholegrain toast spread with 1 tsp margarine and Vegemite

Nutritional Data
Energy & Nutrients: 757 kJ 1809 cal, 243 g carbohydrate, 90 g protein, 56 g fat
Energy Ratio: 52% carbohydrate, 20% protein, 28% fat
Carbohydrate distribution: 79 g breakfast, 68 g lunch, 74 g dinner, 12 g bedtime snack, 12 g from extra milk in beverages.

10000 kJ (2400 cal)

Breakfast
- 1 serve Meg's Muesli topped with 1 sliced banana and 100 mL low-fat milk
- 100 g low-fat fruit yoghurt
- 2 slices wholegrain toast, one spread with 1 tsp margarine and topped with fresh tomato and black pepper, the other with 1 tsp margarine and Date and Fig Spread

Morning Tea
- 1 serve wholegrain biscuits served with 1 tsp margarine

Lunch
- 1 sandwich made with 2 slices pumpernickel bread spread with 2 rounded tsp peanut butter, and filled with chopped celery and lettuce
- 1 sandwich made with 2 slices wholegrain bread each spread with 1 tsp margarine and filled with grated carrot, a sprinkling of sultanas and Creamy Yoghurt Dressing
- 1 apple
- 2 mandarines

Afternoon Tea
- 2 peaches

Dinner
- Orange Borscht (prepared with vegetable stock rather than chicken)
- 1 wholegrain bread roll with 2 tsp margarine
- 1 serve Jumping Bean Bake
- 1 serve Tossed salad
- 1 serve Mocha Mousse
- 1 cup canned apricots (no added sugar)

Bedtime Snack
- 2 slices wholegrain bread topped with 2 x 20 g slices low-fat cheese and grilled

Nutritional Data
Energy & Nutrients: 9995 kJ 2388 cal, 314 g carbohydrate, 116 g protein, 78 g fat
Energy Ratio: 51% carbohydrate, 20% protein, 29% fat
Carbohydrate distribution: 79 g breakfast, 13 g morning tea, 73 g lunch, 14 g afternoon tea, 101 g dinner, 23 g bedtime snack, 12 g from extra milk in beverages.

TIMING YOUR MEALS

To help you control your blood glucose level, you should eat regular meals.

If you're not on medication, in most cases spreading your carbohydrate evenly between 3 meals a day is best.

Make sure that you have three to four serves of high-carbohydrate foods per meal, but the punctuality of mealtimes is not as important as it would be if you were on medication, since you will not be prone to low blood glucose (hypoglycaemia). Avoid eating snacks between meals if you are overweight.

If you're on insulin or diabetes tablets

If you are on medication, then you need to ask what type and when to take it. These questions are best answered in conjunction with your dietitian or diabetes specialist. Find out about your medication so that you can design an eating plan that allows your carbohydrate to be spread in such a way as to keep your blood glucose level within normal range.

An even spread of carbohydrate between three meals daily is usually best, although some people find it easier to regulate blood glucose levels if they eat a carbohydrate-rich snack between meals.

You may find that leaving long gaps between meals, or not eating enough carbohydrate at a meal, may cause your blood glucose level to drop too low (we discuss low blood glucose — hypoglycaemia — on page 42). Also important is the need to **keep your carbohydrate intake even from day to day** to prevent unwanted swings in blood glucose level.

Remember, having diabetes does not affect your need for energy, carbohydrate, protein and fat. It only affects the timing and planning of your meals. On the other hand, your meals and meal pattern must suit your lifestyle, and it may be easier to change the timing and dose of your medication rather than your established eating pattern.

Injected insulin and meals

There are various types of insulin available, classified as short, medium, long-acting, or a combination of these depending on when their activity peaks, and the length of action. Short-acting insulins start to lower your blood glucose level immediately after injection; medium and long-acting insulins may take several hours to begin, and then continue to lower your blood glucose level for several more hours.

The time you eat your carbohydrate should match the activity of your insulin. For instance, if you take a short-acting insulin it is important that you have a carbohydrate-rich meal within 30-40 minutes to prevent hypoglycaemia.

If you have a medium or long-acting insulin in the morning, make sure you have a lunch which is rich in carbohydrate. If you have an injection before your evening meal, the carbohydrate content of your meal and/or supper should be high, depending on the type of insulin.

If your mealtime is delayed, you may have to take a small carbohydrate snack to prevent your blood glucose level dropping too low before you have your next meal.

EATING OUT

Having diabetes does not mean you have to miss out on the good things in life, such as eating out. What it does mean is that you need to understand your diabetes and how to manage it so that you can live the way you want to. Armed with this book and a bit of practice, you will build up the necessary confidence.

Finding your way round the menu

Meals out don't need have to be dull and a few simple changes can make the menu offered at most restaurants fit your needs.

The waiter can tell you what is in dishes if you are unsure.

Because restaurant foods may be high in kilojoules (calories), you would be wise to limit yourself to a starter and main course, or to a main course and fruit dessert.

SOUPS: Thickened and 'creamed' soups will give you carbohydrate, but may be high in fats too. Ask the waiter to leave out the cream. Or ask for a clear soup or a minestrone.

ENTREES (STARTERS): Good choices are fresh oysters, vegetable parcels, skewered meats, seafood on rice, simple salads, asparagus spears or pasta with vegetable sauce.

MAIN COURSES: Select small servings of lean chicken, fish, meat or seafood. Vegetarian and pasta dishes are fine, provided they are not loaded with cream, butter or cheese. To accompany your main course choose pasta, potato or rice to give you plenty of carbohydrate, and other vegetables and salads to add variety, flavour and colour.

BREAD: If the meal you choose does not contain enough carbohydrate, ask for extra bread.

DESSERTS: These are often high in fat, and may contain more sugar than is desirable. If having something sweet to end a meal is important for you, ask for fruit, a simple fruit dessert, a crème caramel or hot soufflé served without cream or rich sauces.

BEVERAGES: Limit your alcohol intake and don't be afraid to ask for a jug of iced water or soda water.

Ethnic Restaurants

Many ethnic restaurants offer good choices. The following ideas may get you started.

Italian:	Minestrone soup. Pasta with a seafood or tomato sauce, plain salad, fruit platter.
Chinese:	Short soup, combination of seafood or meat and vegetables or whole fish in ginger, steamed vegetables, and steamed rice.
Greek:	Dolmades, souvlaki, tabbouleh or green salad without dressing, plain pita bread.
Mexican:	Taco or burritos. Green salad with salsa, refried beans, plain tortillas.
Indian:	Tandoori chicken or fish, riata, vegetable curry, chappatis, plain rice.

Take-away meals

These are often high in fat and salt. The following are better choices in terms of fat:

- Sandwiches, rolls or filled pita bread, hamburger (plain meat and salad), souvlaki, barbecued or char-grilled chicken (no skin), steamed dim sum, hot dog, wholemeal pastie, jacket potatoes (without the sour cream).

Where possible, order some fresh salad or fruit to balance the meal.

Treats and special occasions

Christmas, birthdays and other family get-togethers are especially tempting. If you are the host, choose special recipes from this book for just such occasions. If you are a guest, have a little of the dishes you like, but balance this with vegetables, salad, bread and fruit.

A splurge now and then, on special occasions, does no harm; it's what you do for the rest of the time that counts. Return to your usual eating pattern the next meal. Frequent splurging will contribute to weight gain and poorly controlled diabetes.

TRAVEL

When travelling short distances, try to have your meals at the normal times. When travelling by car, carry dry biscuits, fresh or dried fruits to eat if there are delays.

Overseas travel may mean a change in your normal pattern, particularly when you travel quickly across time zones. It is advisable to notify the airline well in advance and request additional fresh fruit, breads, sandwiches and dry biscuits.

If you are going to cross time zones, discuss your insulin and food requirements with your doctor, dietitian or diabetes educator before you leave on the trip.

When travelling in different countries, you can always find suitable food even if it is limited in variety.

SHIFT WORK

If you are a shift worker, the timing of your meals and medications may vary with the timing of your shifts. Because of the great variation in shifts and individual needs, it is difficult to give suggestions other than strongly advise you to see a dietitian or diabetes educator for help.

Basically you should aim to spread your meals and diabetes medication throughout your waking hours, just as you would on day shift — and treat the day as night. Make sure, if you take your medication prior to going to bed, that you have also eaten.

SPECIAL NEEDS

HYPOGLYCAEMIA

When your blood glucose level drops too low, this is known as hypoglycaemia or 'hypo'. Hypoglycaemia is defined as a blood glucose level below 3.5mmol/litre, and can happen to you if you are on insulin or diabetes tablets. **It does not happen** if you are being treated by diet alone.

How to recognise hypoglycaemia

The symptoms set in quickly. You may experience **one** or **more** of the following:

- Headache
- Dizziness, vagueness
- Extreme hunger
- Blurred vision
- Sweating
- Pins and needles around the mouth
- Paleness, trembling, shaking
- Drowsiness
- Behaviour changes or mood swings (such as bad temper, crying, aggressiveness)

These signs tell you that your blood glucose level may have dropped too low.

Some people who test their blood glucose level regularly may find that their level drops too low without experiencing any symptoms. **If your blood glucose level drops below 3.5 mmol/l, it should be treated as hypoglycaemia whether you have symptoms or not.**

What you should do

Step 1. **Immediately** take sugar to raise your blood glucose level. Any form of sugar will do but the following are recommended as they are quickly absorbed.

- A regular soft drink or Lucozade™ — one glass
- Confectionary such as jelly beans, jubes and life savers — 4-5 lollies
- Sugar in water — about three teaspoons in a cup of water
- Glucodin, powder or tablets, three teaspoons or 2 tablets
- Honey or jam — about one tablespoon.

Do not use low-joule (low-calorie) soft drinks to treat hypoglycaemia.

Step 2. If the symptoms don't improve in five minutes, or become worse, take more sugar as above.

Step 3. If still no improvement in 10 minutes, **contact your doctor or local hospital without delay**.

Step 4. **Always follow the concentrated sugar with a snack of more complex carbohydrate** such as fruit, bread, milk or biscuits, or have your next meal if it is due. This will help prevent your blood glucose level from falling again.

Do not count any extra food taken to treat hypoglycaemia as part of your regular meal plan. Continue with your usual meals.

If not treated **promptly** and **properly**, hypoglycaemia can worsen and lead to unconsciousness. If this happens, others (family, friends, work mates) need to know what to do:

- Roll the person onto their left side. Make sure the airway is clear, tilt the chin up and check the tongue hasn't rolled back.
- Call a doctor or ambulance immediately.
- **Never** give an unconscious person anything to eat or drink.

Medical treatment: The doctor will usually give an injection of a hormone called glucagon which stimulates the liver to release glucose into the bloodstream. Alternatively, he or she may inject a special glucose solution directly into the vein.

It is advisable to carry a small card containing the above information to assist others should you suffer a 'hypo' and become unconscious.

Why it happens

- Taking too much insulin.
- A meal delayed too long.
- Not enough carbohydrate in your food.
- Extra activity (without having extra carbohydrate foods to supply the extra energy — exercise uses your blood glucose supplies).
- Excess alcohol without carbohydrate — such as drinking whisky on an empty stomach.

Simple precautions to prevent hypoglycaemia

- Check your food intake to make sure you are having enough carbohydrate with each meal. If meals are delayed, have some carbohydrate in the form of a snack to tide you over.
- Check your dose of insulin or tablets carefully. Taking too much can make your blood glucose level fall too low.
- If you are more active than usual, you may need extra carbohydrate before, during and after the activity, (*see Exercise, Sport and Diabetes*, page 51).
- If you are drinking alcohol, make sure you eat food containing carbohydrate with it.

Important: If you are having 'hypos' often, consult your doctor to discuss possible causes and solutions. If your diabetes is well controlled, you shouldn't have frequent 'hypos'.

WHAT TO DO IF YOU ARE ILL

If your diabetes is controlled without medication, don't worry if you are unable to eat properly for a day or two. Eat and drink as desired. If you are unwell for longer than this, discuss it with your doctor.

If you are on insulin or diabetes tablets, you must continue with your medication as usual, **no matter how awful you are feeling.** One of the side effects of various illnesses is that your blood glucose level rises, so your medications are absolutely vital to control this. Equally importantly, you must keep on taking carbohydrate even if you are off your food. To do this, try light meals, drinks high in carbohydrate (we've given a number of suitable recipes) or high-carbohydrate snacks. You may find it easier to have a snack or drink every hour, rather than attempt your usual daily meal pattern.

If you are ill for more than two days, or if your blood glucose is consistently higher than 15mmol/litre, contact your doctor.

The following are easy sources of carbohydrate if you are on medication:

- Homemade or canned soup with toast or dry biscuits
- Plain boiled rice or noodles
- Toast or sandwich
- Dry biscuits plain or with thinly sliced cheese, tomato or Vegemite (Promite, Marmite)
- Regular lemonade, dry ginger or other soft drink
- Regular commercially prepared jelly
- Junket
- Creamy rice
- Plain sweet biscuit or cake
- Stewed or canned fruit
- Ice cream
- Milk drinks such as egg flips or Aktavite™ or Milo™
- Fruit juice

If nauseous or vomiting, try sipping drinks such as: dry ginger ale or lemonade, Lucozade™, Staminade™ Enos™, Dexsal™, dry ginger ale or lemonade with ice cream or milk.

Once you can tolerate any of the above, nibble on a dry biscuit or toast, sip chicken noodle soup or try grated apple mixed with a little orange juice.

> *Vomiting or diarrhoea*
>
> *If you are vomiting or suffering from diarrhoea, be aware that it can lead to dehydration and uncontrolled diabetes. You need urgent treatment so contact your doctor right away.*

HIGH BLOOD PRESSURE

Many people with high blood pressure can bring it down by limiting the amount of salt (sodium) in their diet. If overweight, try to reduce your weight as another means of controlling your blood pressure.

If you have high blood pressure you would be wise to:

- Limit the amount of salt you use in cooking
- Avoid adding salt at the table
- Limit the amount of highly salted processed food you eat.

> ### A note about salt
>
> *We have used a little salt where necessary in our recipes. Some dishes simply taste too bland and unappealing without it. However,, we suggest that you always check the flavour of your food before adding salt. Also, remember that in about three weeks you can train your taste buds to appreciate food with less salt, simply by cutting back on the amount of salt you normally eat.*

Here is a list of some of the flavouring agents and processed foods which are high in salt:

- Rock, flavoured and vegetable salts — all of them are salt, no matter what the name
- Monosodium glutamate (MSG or flavour enhancer 621), flavour boosters, meat and vegetable extracts, broth, stock cubes, stock powders and packet soups
- Salted, smoked, cured or pickled meat and fish
- Condiments (sauces), pickles, chutneys, relishes and dressings
- Canned meat, fish and vegetables
- Salted snacks, including potato and corn crisps, nuts and salted biscuits
- Take-away foods such as pizza, barbecued chicken
- Cheese.

Salt substitutes replace all or part of the sodium chloride with potassium chloride. Although these are a satisfactory substitute for ordinary salt, we would prefer you to train your taste buds to enjoy low-salt foods. It is wise to check with your doctor before using these substitutes.

There are many commercial products which are salt-reduced, such as low-salt breads, biscuits, margarines, butters, sauces, canned fish and vegetables. Use them in place of the regular products and learn to read labels. Look out for the words sodium and salt, and for the food additive number 621 as this stands for monosodium glutamate.

Another way in which to give your food zest without using added salt is through herbs and spices. Try adding lemon juice, tomato, onion, garlic, vinegar for extra flavour.

IF YOU HAVE HIGH BLOOD FAT LEVELS (CHOLESTEROL AND TRIGLYCERIDES)

People who have high blood fat levels have an increased risk of heart and blood vessel disease. You run this risk regardless of whether you are overweight or normal weight. The blood fats of concern are cholesterol and triglycerides. Both of these fats are made in the body as well as being provided in foods.

Dietary fats include cholesterol and triglycerides.

Cholesterol is found only in animal products, while triglycerides are found in both animal and vegetable foods.

Foods high in cholesterol include egg yolk, brains, liver, fatty cuts of meat, prawns, squid, fish roe and dairy foods such as cream, butter and cheese.

95 per cent of fat in the diet is in the form of triglycerides. These fats can be categorised as saturated, monounsaturated or polyunsaturated according to their chemical structure. Animal fats are high in saturated fats which may cause a rise in blood fats and contribute to heart disease. Vegetable fats/oils tend to be higher in monounsaturated and polyunsaturated fats which protect against heart disease.

Fats which are highly saturated include those in meats and dairy foods, and the vegetable fats in cocoa butter and coconut.

Fats which are highly unsaturated (monounsaturated or polyunsaturated) include those in seeds, nuts, olives and avocado or oils made from these foods.

> *Note: Saturated Vegetable Fats*
>
> *Be aware that many commercial foods and 'take-aways' contain vegetable fats that have been hydrogenated. This process changes the fats to saturated fats. It is wise to read labels where possible and to limit the use of commercially prepared high fat and fried foods.*

Polyunsaturated and monounsaturated oils and margarines are still high in fats, so they should be used sparingly, particularly if you are overweight.

Although an intake of foods high in fat may increase triglyceride levels, this level can also be raised by alcohol and by eating excessive amounts of refined carbohydrate. High triglyceride levels may also be found in overweight people and in people with undiagnosed or poorly controlled diabetes.

Weight loss and establishing good control of diabetes will help reduce these levels.

Take very seriously our constant reminder to cut down on all fats. Generally, limit all fats and, in particular, animal fats in your diet. See page 20 for 'Hints to help you use less fat'.

If you are concerned about the amount of fat in your diet or require greater detail on the types of fats, consult a dietitian or contact your state division of the National Heart Foundation of Australia.

PREGNANCY AND DIABETES

Diabetes should not stand in the way of a normal, healthy pregnancy. If you have diabetes, make sure that it is under good control where possible before you become pregnant.

You will find that both your nutritional needs and your insulin dosage may need changing while you are pregnant. Get expert help from a dietitian and diabetes specialist and have your diabetes reviewed frequently during your pregnancy so your baby gets the best possible start and you maintain your health throughout.

You may also need to change the timing of your carbohydrate intake at this time, to help with management of your diabetes. **It is particularly important that you eat regular meals, especially breakfast and a bedtime snack.** Long periods without food may increase your risk of ketosis which can be harmful to you and to your baby.

Developing diabetes while pregnant (gestational diabetes)

Some women develop diabetes for the first time during pregnancy, usually after the 26th week. Once the baby is born, the symptoms may disappear, and reappear in later pregnancies. Approximately 50 per cent of women who develop gestational diabetes go on to develop diabetes again in later life.

To ensure that you and your baby are healthy, once you have been diagnosed as having diabetes, you must take particular care of your diet throughout the remainder of your pregnancy. This is usually all that is needed to control your blood glucose level.

Furthermore, if you control your weight from then on, and make sure your diet is low in fats and added sugars, while high in complex carbohydrate and fibre, you can help prevent or delay the onset of diabetes in later life. This underscores an important point: **good nutrition and keeping slim are two of your best protections** against developing diabetes.

CHILDREN AND ADOLESCENTS

You will find the guidelines set out in this book will ensure that children and adolescents with diabetes enjoy the benefits of up-to-date dietary management.

Just as their insulin requirements will vary, so will their dietary needs; it is a good idea to have your child or adolescent's diet reviewed at least annually by a dietitian, and their diabetes and general health monitored regularly. However, do remember that for children and adolescents, food has important social implications. While instilling in your child or adolescent enjoyment of a healthy eating plan, you may have to compromise at times. Food and eating should not become a battlefield, a focus of rebellion or a source of family tension. To begin with, the entire family would benefit by eating in exactly the same way. This takes away any sense of 'being different' or being deprived.

There is a common misconception that the food you should prepare for your offspring with diabetes is by its very nature unpalatable and 'unusual'. The menu plans and recipes in this book show just how unnecessary and wrong this view is; teach all your children about a varied and balanced eating plan, encourage a liking for cereals, vegetables and fruit, and you will have achieved something of lifelong value.

Be flexible and make an effort in the kitchen to prepare food that delights and satisfies. Remember, too, that children and adolescents like to snack, so prepare healthy and delicious ones in advance so that you don't hear the complaint 'There's nothing to eat', meaning 'There is nothing ready prepared which I can pick up in my fingers right away.' This avoids problems where children and adolescents turn to fast foods and processed products because they are so easy to get hold of. Providing alternatives is half the battle; good sense will see you through the rest.

Tips and traps for children and adolescents

- With young children, it is important that they take an active part in their diabetes management, including blood glucose monitoring, their insulin injections, food choices and planning their meals. You will find that the more involved your child is, the less tension is likely to arise.

- Avoid making diabetes the focus of family life; it's just one aspect. Don't force your child to eat; you don't always feel hungry, neither do they. Forcing a reluctant child to eat leads to resentment, rebellion and anxiety for everyone. It's totally counter-productive. You may find, in the name of co-operation and family well-being, that you have to sometimes make a temporary compromise on diabetes control for the sake of long-term outcome.

- By learning to monitor their own blood glucose level, your child will soon learn the effects different foods have on it.

- Teach your children the benefits of regular meals and a healthy way of eating. It's an investment in their future health. Use this approach and your child will come to see healthy eating as a positive aspect of life rather than as a negative aspect of having diabetes. Children (and adults for that matter) should learn that diabetes does not mean being punished or deprived of food.

- It's easy to fall into the trap of replacing uneaten vegetables and cereals with sugary foods because of a fear of hypoglycaemia. Children are smart and they will soon learn to manipulate; they may start refusing their meals knowing you may offer them a sweet treat instead. Try offering healthier alternatives in this situation: fruit, milk or dry biscuits will do the trick.

- Encourage your child to carry extra snacks, especially when they will be away from home for long periods such as sleeping out on weekends or going to after-school activities.

- Make sure parents of friends, and teachers at school, know that your child has diabetes and that they know how to cope with hypoglycaemia and sickness.

- Let your child know that there are other children with diabetes. They are neither alone nor unique. Diabetes camps are an excellent way to reduce any sense of isolation. For details of these camps, get in touch with DIABETES AUSTRALIA or the local children's hospital.

Foreground: curry accompaniments – Fresh Mango Chutney, low-fat yoghurt and Riata – beside mountain bread. Centre left: Vegetable Curry and right, Beef Curry served with steamed brown rice and Moong Dahl (at the top).

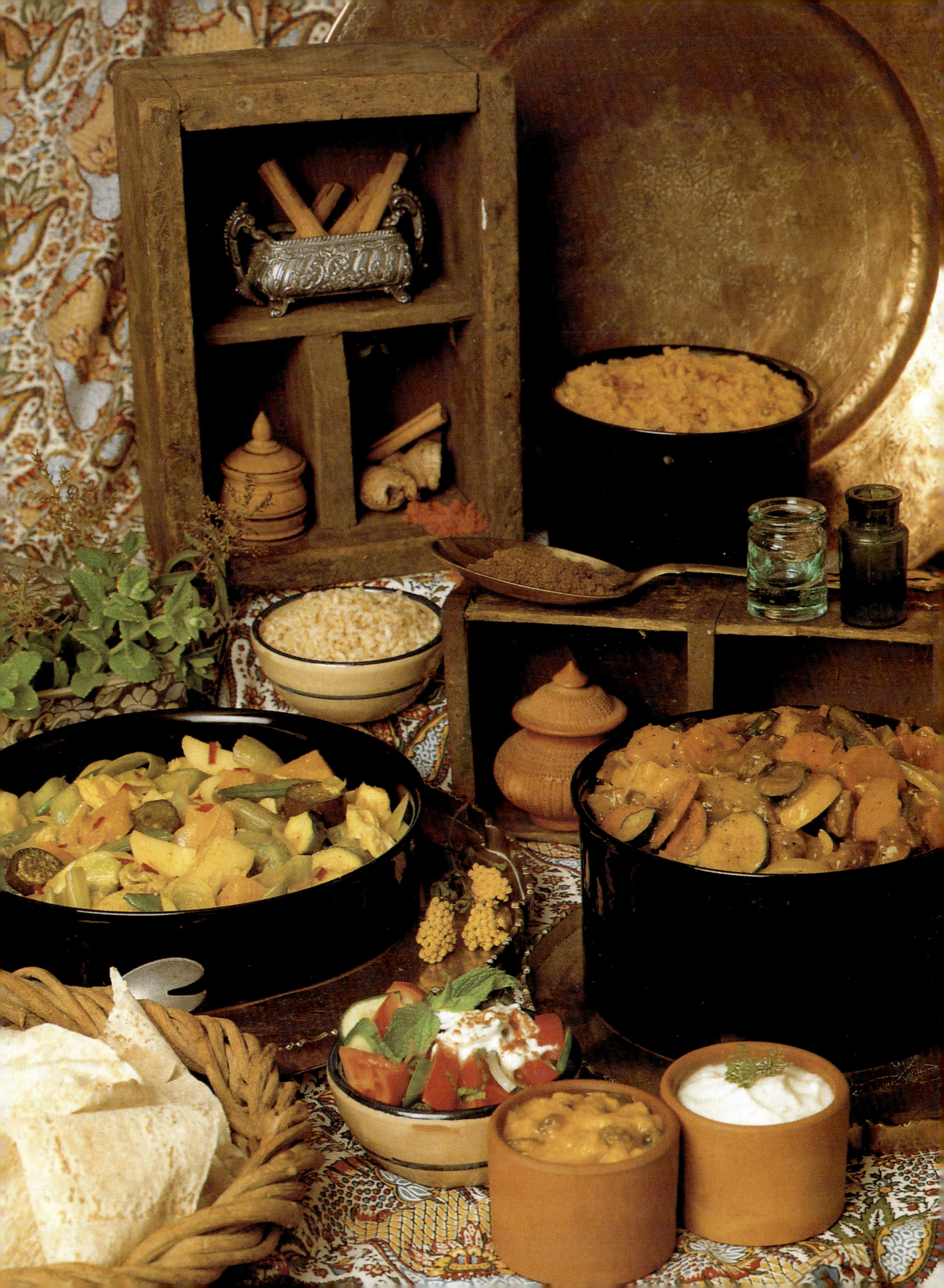

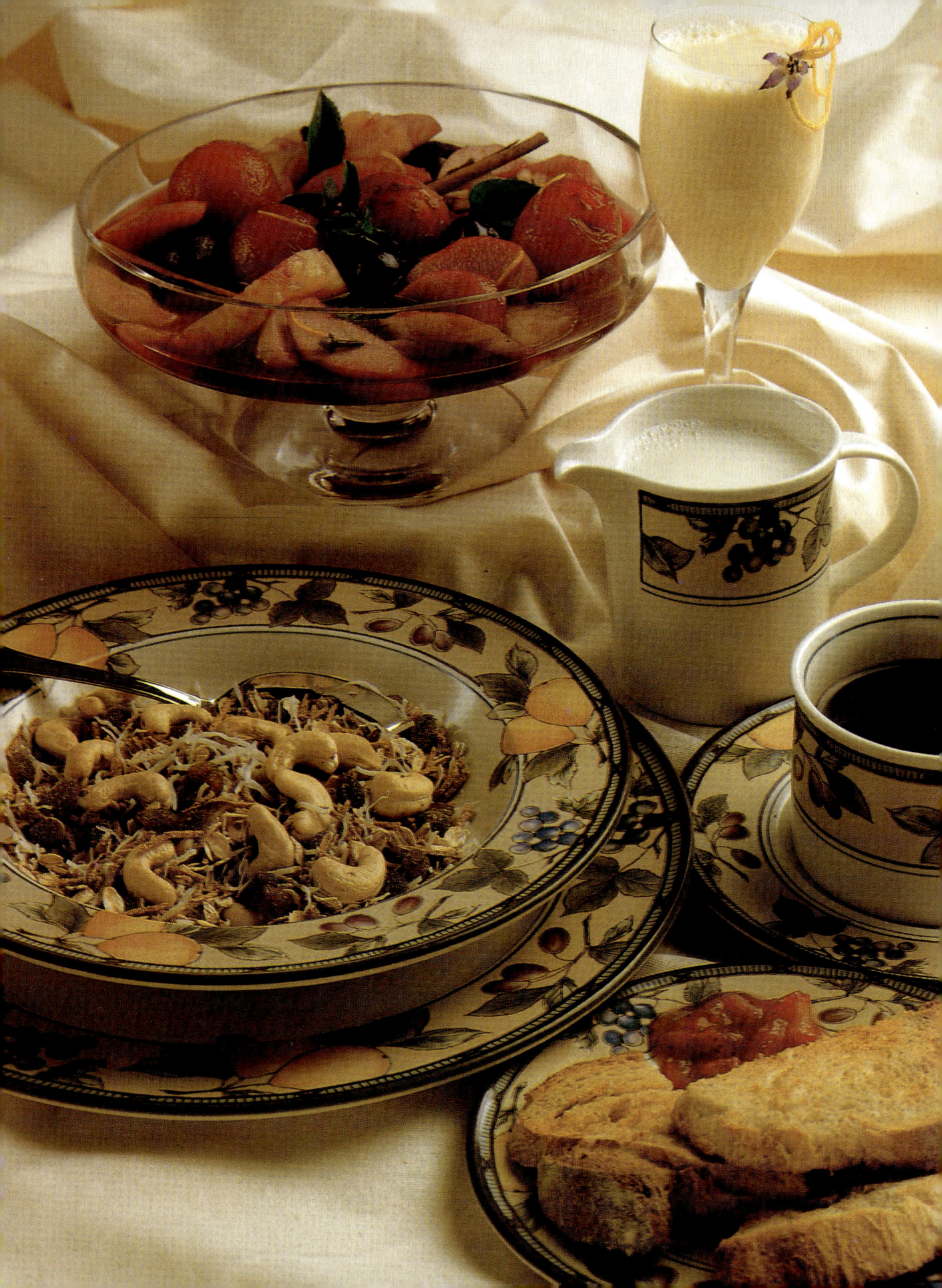

- Diabetes is not a barrier to normal childhood activities such as parties, sport, staying at friends', trips or school camps, and you should encourage your child to take part.

- The better your child understands his or her diabetes, the more responsibility they will take for it and so they will cope better with their own changing needs as they grow older.

- Don't turn your child into a 'cupboard eater' or 'food sneak' by never letting them taste sweet foods. That old phrase, 'moderation in all things' holds good. You may well find that denying your child any sweet foods leads to secret eating and binges. Simply don't make a fuss about fatty or sweet foods; remember that the occasional splurge will not cause any long-term harm.

- Adolescence brings its own special needs. The teens are a time of exploration, testing and a desire or need for independence. This applies to the issue of food just as much as it does to other realms of behaviour. If your teenager has a good knowledge of diabetes management, they will know how to be flexible in terms of mealtimes, foods eaten, the amount of insulin they need and when they need it. This may cause you considerable anxiety, but you must learn to encourage your child's sense of independence; allow them to learn by their own mistakes.

- For adolescents, the peer pressure to drink alcohol may be strong. Make sure your teenager understands how vital it is for them to have plenty of carbohydrate when they drink alcohol.

- Adolescents also need to realise **how vital it is to seek medical help the moment they do not feel well.** Failure to do this is a common cause of hospital admissions for uncontrolled diabetes.

- Hormonal changes and growth spurts during adolescence may upset your adolescents' diabetes control even though they are doing the right thing. It may be that their whole management routine needs a fresh appraisal.

VEGETARIANS WITH DIABETES

The guidelines in this book are ideal for people who are vegetarian. Many of the recipes have been created with vegetarians in mind, and on pages 37–38 you will find vegetarian meal plans showing how to balance your nutritional needs.

You can follow a vegetarian diet, be well nourished and keep your diabetes under control. But you should to be aware that as a vegetarian you can miss out on some nutrients. It is therefore vital that you know how to plan your diet to ensure these are included in adequate amounts.

To begin with, we suggest that you include dairy products and eggs in your vegetarian eating plan (in other words, what is termed 'lacto-ovo vegetarian'). However, if you choose out of matters of conscience or religion to follow a strict vegan lifestyle (in other words, do not eat any animal products at all), we strongly recommend that you consult a dietitian, who will help you plan an adequate diet.

The principles in this book apply to vegetarians; however there are other tips which are particularly important.

Toast and Strawberry Conserve, a bowl of Meg's Muesli with a lavish sprinkling of cashew nuts, English Fruit Compote and, at the back, a refreshing glass of Orange Buttermilk.

Tips and traps for vegetarians:

- The nutrients that may be lacking in a poorly planned diet are: iron, zinc, protein, calcium, cyanocobalamin (Vitamin B12) and riboflavin (B2).

- The best sources of iron and zinc for vegetarians are pulses, wholegrain cereal products, green leafy vegetables and eggs. However, these foods do not release their minerals into your system as readily as do animal sources, such as meat.

- To increase your absorption of iron from non-meat sources include foods with Vitamin C at the same meal. For instance, include citrus fruits, pineapple, tomatoes or juice made from them when you eat iron-rich food such as cereal products, spinach or silverbeet.

- The tannin in tea interferes with the absorption of iron into your body, so don't finish your meal with a cup of tea.

- Fibre slows the absorption of vitamins and minerals in your digestive tract, so you may have to eat more of certain foods to counter this.

- Eat the recommended daily amounts of dairy products and eggs set out below, to ensure your protein, calcium, cyanocobalamin (B12) and riboflavin (B2) needs are met.

A Guide to Recommended Daily Food Intake for Lacto-Ovo Vegetarians

Milk and dairy products

600 mL (1 pint) milk or the equivalent in cheese and/or yoghurt

1 cup milk = 30 g (1 oz) hard cheese
         = 1 cup yoghurt

Note: Low-fat cheeses such as cottage and ricotta are poor sources of calcium.

Other protein-rich foods

We recommend that you eat two serves of the following every day:

- eggs
- pulses
- nuts
- soy bean curd (tofu)

- 1 serve = 2
- 1 serve = 3/4 cup
- 1 serve = 90 g (3 oz)
- 1 serve = 1 cup (220 g or 7 oz)

Note: Because vegetarian diets are generally low in high cholesterol foods, don't worry about limiting your intake of eggs.

Guidelines for other foods

Make sure that your daily diet also includes:

Fruits	At least two to three serves
Vegetables	At least five serves
Bread and cereals	A minimum of four serves or more, according to appetite
Fats	1-2 tablespoons, including some table margarine

Tips for vegans

- Suitable protein sources include **fortified soya milk**, pulses, nuts, seeds and cereal products. As the protein quality from these sources is not as good as animal sources, you need to eat a variety of these products every day.

- Alternative cyanocobalamin (B12) sources include **fortified soya milk** (check the label). As only a few milks are fortified, a supplement is recommended.

- Alternative calcium sources include **fortified soya milk** (check the label). Sesame and sunflower seeds, tahine and almonds contain small amounts of calcium.

- Alternative riboflavin (B2) sources include **fortified soya milk** (check the label), Vegemite, dried fruits, pulses, nuts and green leafy vegetables.

> *A note about soya milk and diabetes*
>
> *Many brands of soya milk have added sugar (usually in the form of sucrose). This is also common in flavoured soya milk, so we advise you to read the labels. Regular soya milks are poor sources of calcium, riboflavin (B2) and cyanocobalamin (B12).*

EXERCISE, SPORT AND DIABETES

Regular exercise is important for everyone who wants to achieve and maintain good health. This means at least 30 minutes three times a week. Good forms of exercise include brisk walking, swimming, bike riding or aerobics. To know whether your body is benefiting from exercise, check your pulse immediately afterwards; it should be faster than your usual resting level.

For people with diabetes, exercise has another function: it helps people with diabetes keep their blood glucose level within normal range. People with **non-insulin dependent diabetes** can improve the control of their diabetes and minimise their need for medication by exercising or playing sport regularly.

If you have insulin-dependent diabetes, regular exercise is important, but requires more careful planning. You will learn from experience how your body reacts to exercise and how best to balance your energy expenditure with the needs of your diabetes.

EXERCISE AND YOUR BLOOD GLUCOSE LEVEL
For the person without diabetes

The body is able to keep blood glucose level constant during sport through the release of insulin and other hormones.

When exercise begins, the body normally stops releasing insulin and produces the hormones adrenalin and glucagon which stimulate the liver to release glucose into the blood. The insulin already present in the bloodstream allows the exercising muscles to take up the glucose, converting it to energy and keeping the blood glucose level constant.

As the exercise continues, the blood glucose level normally goes up and the liver then stops releasing glucose. Now the body releases insulin again, so that more glucose can pass into the exercising muscle. This complex mechanism ensures that the blood glucose level normally remains constant.

What happens if you have insulin-dependent diabetes?

If you have insulin-dependent diabetes, you don't have the benefit of this natural control. Once you have taken your insulin injection, you cannot regulate its action. This means that you may have a wide variation in your blood glucose level during and after exercise. However, **if you have enough insulin** in your system and your blood glucose level is within the normal range at the start of exercise, then you can safely exercise.

If you don't have enough insulin available in your system when you begin exercising — in other words, your blood glucose level is high — your body can misread the situation and release more glucose into your bloodstream from the liver. Because you don't have enough insulin, the glucose can't pass into your muscle cells. As a result, your blood glucose level will rise excessively (hyperglycaemia). So check your glucose levels before you begin. **You shouldn't exercise if your blood glucose is above 16 mmol/l.**

If, on the other hand, you have too much insulin in your blood and your blood glucose level is low, your liver shuts down its release of glucose. The insulin continues to carry glucose to your muscles, leading to a rapid fall in your blood glucose level (hypoglycaemia). In this case take more carbohydrate before you begin to exercise.

Tips and Traps

Hypoglycaemia is the most common concern for people on diabetes medication who exercise regularly. However, there are some simple steps you can take to help prevent this problem.

- Where possible, check your blood glucose level before you exercise, especially if you are new to diabetes. If you feel your level is low, then take a carbohydrate snack before you begin exercising. You may find it useful to take another test after the exercise or during it if it is prolonged, so you become familiar with the effect exercise has on your blood glucose level.

- If you are exercising away from home, make sure you have some carbohydrate foods with you, such as fruit, fruit juice, barley sugar or biscuits.

- If you have been doing vigorous exercise, your blood glucose level may continue to drop after you stop exercising, so you should eat some carbohydrate afterwards, too.

- Be aware of dehydration. But don't confuse this with hypoglycaemia which relates not to fluids but to blood glucose level. If you exercise vigorously and especially in hot weather, **keep drinking plenty of fluids before, during and after you exercise.**

- When your exercise session is over, quench your thirst with a non-alcoholic drink. Alcohol may lower your blood glucose level further and also has a dehydrating effect.

- Serious athletes with diabetes (and there are many) ensure that their diabetes is well controlled before they begin training. Training is the time to fine tune control. They know that this will ensure peak performance during competition.

How to adjust your food intake

Once your diabetes is controlled, you will need to learn how to manipulate the balance between food, insulin and activity. The only way to do this properly is to monitor your blood glucose level before, during and after you exercise and experiment until you are confident about the combination which suits your needs best.

Use this ready-reckoner as a starting point to work out your carbohydrate intake and adjust it to suit your individual needs.

Activity	Time	Blood Glucose Level prior to activity (mmol/l)	Recommended additional carbohydrate intake
Low Level	½ hour	< 5.5	15 g CHO (one serve fruit, bread, biscuit, yoghurt or milk)
		> 5.6	No extra food
Moderate Intensity	1 hour	< 5.5	20-30 g CHO (1½–2 serves fruit, bread, biscuits, yoghurt and/or milk).
		5.6–10	15 g CHO (one serve fruit, bread, biscuit, yoghurt or milk).
		10–16	No extra food (in most cases).
		> 16	No extra food. Exercise not recommended: blood glucose level may go up.
Strenuous Activity	1–2 hours	< 5.5	45-60 g CHO (1 sandwich and fruit and/or milk or yoghurt).
		5.6–10	25-50 g CHO (1 sandwich and fruit and/or milk or yoghurt).
		10–16	15 g CHO (1 serve fruit, bread, biscuits, yoghurt or milk).
		> 16	Exercise not recommended: blood glucose level may go up.
Varying Intensity	Long Duration ½–1 day		Insulin may best be decreased. (Conservatively decrease the insulin dose due to peak at time of activity by 10%. A 50% reduction is not uncommon.)
			Increase CHO before, during and after activity.
			15–50 g CHO per hour, such as diluted fruit juice, or sports drinks.

CHO=Carbohydrate

HOW TO MODIFY RECIPES

Some of your old family favourite recipes may seem unsuitable if you have diabetes. Before putting them away, see if you can alter them to suit your new eating pattern. You may be able to reduce the fat and sugar, and increase the fibre without changing the flavour or appearance of the dish very much, if at all.

We have taken a typical family dish to show you how to adapt it. *The changes in ingredients and method are shown in italics.*

Bread and Butter Pudding

4 thin slices bread	*Use wholemeal bread*
4 tbsp sugar	*Use an alternative sweetener or 1 tbsp sugar and vanilla essence for more flavour*
½ cup raisins	
2 tbsp butter	*3 tsp should be enough and use polyunsaturated margarine*
2 eggs	
500 mL (1 pt) milk	*Use low-fat milk*

1. Grease a pie dish.

    No need to grease.

2. Spread the bread with butter (*margarine*) and layer it in the dish with sugar and raisins sprinkled in between.

    Use far less sugar or if you prefer a sweet pudding, add sweetener to the eggs and milk.

3. Beat the eggs and milk.

    Add sweetener and vanilla if preferred to sugar.

4. Pour egg mixture over the bread and leave to stand for 10 minutes. Then bake in moderate oven until the custard is set, approximately 20-25 minutes.

Tips and traps in modifying recipes

MAIN DISHES

- Consider whether you can cut down on the amount of meat. 120 grams (4 oz) per person is sufficient. This means 500 grams (1 lb) should feed four.
- Choose lean cuts and trim off any visible fat.
- If bacon is used as a flavouring, try using a little lean ham, ham bone or bacon stock cube instead — in which case you will not need to add more salt.
- Reduce fats. For browning foods, use a non-stick pan over high heat to dry-fry foods such as meat. Alternatively, use a cooking spray or a pastry brush to brush a thin layer of oil on the base of the pan — you really need very little to do the trick.
- Don't use more than 2 teaspoons of added fat for a recipe serving four, or leave out the fat if you can.
- If a recipe uses cream or sour cream as a sauce, you can often use non-fat yoghurt instead, but remember to add it at the last minute and not allow the sauce to reboil or the yoghurt will curdle.
- For white sauces, use low-fat or skim milk in place of full cream milk. Use the minimum amount of butter or margarine, or use cornflour (cornstarch) with low-fat milk and don't use fat at all.
- To add fibre and decrease the meat, include some dried beans or lentils in mixed dishes with meat. This works wonderfully in pasta sauces, lasagne, curries and casseroles.

DESSERTS AND CAKES

Many of these recipes modify well, so try your old standbys with a few changes, such as:

- Substitute wholemeal flour for white, or, if the result is too heavy, use a half-and-half mixture.
- If you substitute wholemeal flour in a recipe, you usually have to add a little more liquid to get a moist result.
- Substitute skim or low-fat milk for full cream milk.
- Reduce or remove the butter or margarine. Where a recipe specifies that you cream butter and sugar, minimise the sugar, reduce the butter and rub into the dry ingredients.
- Where you have reduced butter and sugar in a recipe, it will not rise as high, and the texture will be a little denser. Try using a smaller baking tin.

And if your recipe can't be modified . . .

Some recipes simply don't look and taste the same if modified. Put these on your list of occasional dishes and keep them as treats — and then only have a small serve.

PLEASURES OF THE TABLE

Using the recipes in this book

Most of the recipes in this book are simple and quick to prepare. In most cases, we avoid using unusual ingredients, although we slip some in, now and again, to encourage you to experiment.

Flavour: You can increase or decrease the flavour intensity of recipes to suit your own taste. Experiment with herbs and spices; cut back or add more as you like. Such flavour enhancers will not alter the nutritional value of your food.

If microwaving any of the dishes, you may need to increase the amount of herbs and spices we recommend because microwaving does not always allow for the flavours to develop and combine.

Salt: We follow the good health guideline of 'cut back on salt'. However, we use common sense, and where we feel that a recipe needs a little salt we add it or use soy sauce or stock cubes.

We encourage you to minimise or omit salt wherever possible. Where we refer to soy sauce in the recipes, we suggest you use light or salt-reduced soy sauce.

Sugar: We use a variety of sweetening agents in our recipes, including sugar in small amounts. There are good reasons for this. Firstly, we now know that a small amount of sugar taken in a mixed meal or recipe does not cause a significant rise in the blood glucose level. Secondly, some recipes, especially baked products, rely on sugar to produce good results. Thirdly, there are some instances where the flavour of sugar is superior to that of artificial sweeteners — it does not alter or lose taste during the cooking process.

You will also see that we use natural sweetening agents other than sucrose (table sugar), such as fruit juice, dried fruits and fruit juice concentrates, with delicious results.

A range of artificial sweeteners are also used.

Fat: We use a number of ways to reduce the fat content of our recipes. For example, we frequently sauté using water or a hot dry pan instead of oil. Where oil is used we have kept it to a minimum by recommending that you brush the frying pan with oil rather than pouring it in.

Generally we use skim or low-fat milk (1.5-2% fat). Likewise, with yoghurt; in most cases, you can substitute low-fat natural yoghurt for full cream yoghurt. But not always: for instance, full-cream yoghurt is absolutely necessary in Quick Wholemeal Bread (recipe, page 191).

Where we use cottage cheese, it is always the skim milk variety; ricotta cheese is always low-fat ricotta; low-fat block cheese is cheese of less than 17% fat. Low-fat cream cheese is a mixture of approximately half and half cottage and cream cheese where you mix your own, or the commercial variety of less than 17% fat. To enhance the flavour of some recipes, we include a small amount of higher fat tasty cheeses, such as parmesan. Here, we use the principle that a small amount goes a long way.

Fibre: We use wholemeal products as much as possible. However, there are times when the texture or flavour of the dish is better with a mixture of wholegrain and refined flours or cereals. In a few recipes, we use the refined product only to give a more traditional result. Using wholemeal flour products gives a heavier or denser texture than white flour, and requires more liquid during cooking. We allow for this in our recipes.

When using the oven: Always turn your oven on in plenty of time so it is at the correct temperature when you are ready to bake.

Analysis: Where a choice of ingredients is given in a recipe, the first one listed is the one we use in our analysis of nutritional value.

Breakfasts

For a good start to a great day, make sure you have breakfast. We've given ideas from leisurely Sunday breakfasts through to simple quick ideas for the weekday rush. Breakfast can be as simple as a bowl of cereal and a serve of fruit, or as beguiling as a fruit platter followed by mouthwatering pancakes.

Start your day with plenty of carbohydrate and fibre. Begin with a breakfast cereal. This can be homemade or you can choose from the excellent commercial products available (see page 30). Porridge makes a terrific start to the day and lends itself to interesting toppings such as sultanas, diced raw apple, cinnamon or nuts.

Make your own breakfast blend using: oats, all-bran; wheatgerm; bran (all sorts – rice, corn, oat, barley or wheat); dried fruits of every kind; unsalted raw nuts; seeds (pumpkin, sesame, linseed and sunflower); millet; buckwheat; puffed rice, wheat or corn; and wheatflakes. Serve with hot or cold skim or low-fat milk, yoghurt and fruit.

With toast or bread, look at the toppings and fillings suggested on page 62. Consider the recipes for Date and Fig Spread, Strawberry Spread, and Dried Apricot Conserve in this section.

Fruit cleanses the palate and provides vitamins and minerals as well as carbohydrate and fibre. Eat it fresh, stewed or canned without added sugar. Combine fruits, top them with low-fat yoghurt, cottage or ricotta cheese, or add them to porridge, cereal, or eat them on their own.

Cooked breakfasts are a pleasant treat. They need not take long to prepare. Try:

- Baked beans with freshly chopped mushrooms or capsicum (green pepper)
- Tomatoes, asparagus, mushrooms or sweetcorn on toast
- Poached, scrambled or boiled eggs
- Omelettes with fillings such as low-fat cheese and herbs, tomato combined with lean ham and onion, or a mushroom sauce

Meg's Muesli

Makes: approximately 1 kg (2.2 lb)

4 cups rolled oats or barley
2 cups shredded coconut
1 cup sultanas
1 cup unsalted cashews, chopped
2 cups unprocessed bran
2 cups all-bran
1½ cups wheatgerm

You can develop your own muesli recipe according to taste, but be very careful about the ingredients you add — check them against the ready reckoner at the end of this book to find out whether the additional ingredients you want to use have more fat than we recommend. Watch out, too, for added sugar.

Method:

Mix all ingredients well with a large spoon or your fingers.

Allow ⅓ cup per serve.

Nutritional data per serve: 470 kJ (112 cal), CHO 12 g, Protein 4 g, Fat 6 g.

Preparation time: 15 minutes.

Liquid Breakfast

Serves: 4

2 cups skim or low-fat milk
1 cup low-fat natural yoghurt
3 ripe bananas or 1 cup fresh strawberries or unsweetened canned peaches or apricots
2 eggs (optional)
Equal™ or other artificial sweetener, to taste
garnish: ground allspice, cinnamon or nutmeg

If you simply don't have a moment in the mornings, this quick breakfast comes in a glass.

Method:

1. Place all ingredients in a blender or food processor and blend well.
2. Serve at once, topped with a sprinkling of spice.

Nutrition data per serve: 749 kJ (179 cal), CHO 26 g, Protein 12 g, Fat 4 g.

Preparation time: 5 minutes. Equipment: food processor or blender.

Coddled Egg

Serves: 1

1 egg
1 slice wholemeal bread
½ tsp margarine
pepper
pinch salt

Method:

1. Bring water to boil in saucepan, lower egg in gently and soft boil to preference (3-5 minutes).
2. Crumble bread into an individual serving bowl.
3. Add margarine, pepper and salt.
4. Lift egg out of water, crack open top, and spoon soft egg onto bread mixture.
5. Stir together gently and serve.

To vary: add ½ tsp of finely chopped chives or parsley at step 3.

Nutrition data per serve: 607 kJ (145 cal), CHO 10 g, Protein 8 g, Fat 8 g.
Preparation time: 10 minutes. Cooking equipment: small saucepan.

Fresh Strawberry Conserve

Makes: 1 cup

1 punnet strawberries, hulled and roughly chopped
1 tbsp water
1 tbsp lemon juice
1 level tsp gelatine soaked in 1½ tbsp water
2 sachets Equal™ or other artificial sweetener equivalent to 4 level tsp sugar

You can vary this recipe by using other berries instead of strawberries.

Method:

1. Place strawberries in saucepan with water and lemon juice.
2. Cover, bring to boil and simmer for 10 minutes, or microwave on 'high' for 5 minutes.
3. Mash fruit slightly and stand for 10 minutes.
4. Dissolve gelatine according to instructions on packet, and add to fruit.
5. Stir in sweetener.
6. Pour into a clean hot jar. Cover, cool and refrigerate.

To store: refrigerate for up to two weeks.

Nutrition data per total quantity: 168 kJ (40 cal), CHO 6 g, Protein 4 g, Fat trace.
Preparation time: 30 minutes. Cooking equipment: small saucepan.

Date and Fig Spread

Makes: 2 cups

1 cup seedless dates
1 cup dried figs
6 tsp lemon juice
¼ cup orange juice

The dates and figs have all the sweetness you need as a substitute for traditional sugar-laden jams.

Method:

1. Chop fruit finely.
2. Add to bowl, pour juice over, cover and soak overnight.
3. Spoon into blender or food processor and blend for approximately 2 minutes until smooth.
4. Store, covered, in a jar in refrigerator.

To store: cover and refrigerate up to two weeks.

Nutrition data per total quantity: 3312 kJ (791 cal), CHO 196 g, Protein 10 g, Fat trace.
Preparation time: 15 minutes plus overnight soaking. Cooking equipment: food processor or blender.

Dried Apricot Conserve

Makes: 1 cup

1 cup dried apricots
juice of 1 orange
pinch cinnamon
pinch ground cloves
½ cup warm water

You can vary this delectable yet simple recipe by using a dried fruit medley, dried peaches or dried pears. You can also replace the cloves with fresh or ground ginger.

Method:

1. Chop apricots roughly.
2. Combine in mixing bowl with juice, spices, and water. Cover. Allow to stand 1 hour.
3. Spoon into saucepan and cook gently for approximately 10 minutes over low heat, stirring constantly, until mixture thickens and starts to combine. Alternatively, spoon into a bowl and microwave on 'high' for 5 minutes. Stir two or three times during cooking until mixture thickens and starts to combine.
4. Spoon into container, cover and cool.
5. Stir again, adding a little more water if necessary, then refrigerate until ready to use.

To store: cover and refrigerate for up to two weeks.

Nutrition data per total quantity: 1248 kJ (298 cal), CHO 69 g, Protein 8 g, Fat trace.
Preparation time: 1½ hours. Cooking equipment: small saucepan or microwave dish.

Appetisers and Snacks

Here we give you some ideas for quick and light meals, cocktail parties and pre-dinner hors d'oeuvres. Remember the basic principles of low fat when planning appetisers and snacks. The recipes in this section are also a useful source of carbohydrate which you can use to balance your daily meal plan.

If you are overweight, be careful not to over-indulge in these tempters.

Bread, pumpernickel or wholemeal biscuits make a good base for appetisers. Here are a few ideas:

Accompaniments for dips

Vegetables: carrot sticks, cauliflower and broccoli florets, celery sticks, cucumber wedges, green or red capsicum (bell pepper) pieces, mushroom (button or slices), radish wedges, spring onions (shallots).

Fruits: apple wedges tossed in lemon juice to prevent browning, rock melon (cantaloupe) or honey dew melon cut into chunks, kiwifruit wedges, fresh pineapple pieces, pear slices, fresh apricot halves.

Bread and biscuits: crusty wholemeal bread, dark rye or pumpernickel slices, triangles of toast or zweibach, pita bread triangles (fresh or toasted), plain dry biscuits, crispbread or rusks.

Asparagus Rolls:

To serve four, you will need three slices of wholemeal bread and three slices of white high-fibre bread. Cut off the crusts, roll the bread to flatten it a little, spread with margarine very lightly and place a spear of cooked fresh asparagus or canned asparagus diagonally across each slice of bread. Roll the bread towards a corner, press lightly to seal the edges of the bread. Cut each in half. Finally, garnish with rings of green or red capsicum (bell pepper) and parsley.

Pumpernickel Savouries:

Many different combinations can be used to top rounds or squares of pumpernickel to make interesting and tasty savouries. Try these ideas:

- Baby prawns or shrimps and avocado
- Smoked salmon slices or rolls garnished with capers
- Sliced hard-boiled egg topped with black caviar and tiny sprigs of parsley
- Circles or squares of lean ham with asparagus tips
- Low-fat cottage cheese topped with strawberry halves or slices of peach or nectarine

Sandwich Fillings

Remember when you use any of these delicious fillings you do not need to use margarine on the bread — and use wholemeal bread rather than white. Use fillings for jaffles or open sandwiches.

Cheese and . . .

- A mixture of grated low-fat block cheese, grated apple, carrot, chopped celery and pecans or walnuts; bind with Creamy Yoghurt Dressing (recipe, page 160)
- Ricotta cheese with sliced cucumber, tomato and chopped basil
- Ricotta cheese with chopped celery and walnuts
- Mustard, grated low-fat block cheese and sliced olives
- Sliced low-fat block cheese, thinly sliced green apple and Fresh Mango Pickle (recipe, page 163)

Fish and . . .

- Salmon or tuna in brine, with sliced cucumber or celery, topped with Creamy Yoghurt Dressing (recipe, page 160)
- Shrimp, ricotta cheese and thinly sliced cucumber
- Smoked salmon, low-fat cream cheese and capers

Meat or Chicken and . . .

- Fresh Mango Pickle (recipe, page 163) or mustard topped with thinly sliced cold lean meat
- Chopped chicken, chives and parsley bound with Creamy Yoghurt Dressing (recipe page 160)
- Chopped chicken, walnuts and celery or green capsicum (bell pepper), bound with low-fat natural yoghurt
- Whole seed mustard, chopped lean ham and grated apple
- Chopped chicken topped with thinly sliced raw mushrooms and Curry Dressing (recipe, page 161)

Egg and . . .

- Scrambled eggs with finely chopped lean ham
- Hard-boiled eggs mashed with alfalfa or bean sprouts and Curry Dressing (recipe, page 161)

Vegetables and . . .

- Canned baked beans, lightly mashed and seasoned with tabasco sauce
- Peanut butter and sliced cucumber or chopped celery
- Mashed kidney or three-bean mix with chilli, capsicum (bell pepper), cucumber and onion

Sweet Fillings and . . .

- Mashed banana, lemon juice and cinnamon
- Cottage or ricotta cheese with chopped dried figs

Chicken Liver Pâté

Serves: 6 as an appetiser

250 g (8 oz) chicken livers
¼ cup water
1 sprig fresh or ¼ tsp dried thyme
2 bay leaves
coarsely ground black pepper to taste
salt to taste
½ cup port
garnish: coarsely ground black pepper

Chicken liver pâté is usually made with lashings of butter and cream. This recipe avoids additional fats, yet tastes delicious.

Method:

1. Wash, dry and roughly chop the livers, discarding any greenish portions (these are not a sign of deterioration, but may discolour the pâté).
2. In saucepan, bring water to the boil. Add the liver and stir until sealed, about 2 minutes.
3. Add the thyme, bay leaves, pepper and salt. Cover, reduce heat and simmer gently for 10 minutes.
4. Add port and simmer, uncovered, a further 3 minutes.
5. If using fresh thyme, remove and discard the sprig. Remove and discard bay leaves.
6. Allow mixture to cool slightly. Purée liver and cooking liquids in a food processor or blender.

To vary: replace port with 4 tbsp each of orange juice and brandy and add the grated rind of half an orange.

To store: cover and refrigerate for up to three days.

To serve — As an appetiser: spoon the pâté into a serving bowl, sprinkle with black pepper, and chill for at least 1 hour before serving. Surround the dip with sliced fresh vegetables, biscuits or triangles of dry toast.

As an entrée: spoon the pâté into small, individual pots or ramekins. Smooth over the surface, sprinkle with black pepper and chill for at least 1 hour before serving. Place the pots on small plates and arrange a couple of dry toast triangles or crisp biscuits on each plate.

Nutrition data per serve (6 serves as appetiser): kJ 410.2 (98 cal), CHO 3 g, Protein 9 g, Fat 3 g.

Preparation time: 30 minutes. Cooking equipment: heavy-based saucepan, food processor or blender.

Moong Dhal

Makes: 2 cups

1 cup dried red lentils
3 cups water
½ tsp turmeric
1 tomato, peeled and chopped
2 tsp oil
½ tsp cumin seeds
3 curry leaves (optional)
1 onion, finely chopped or minced
2 cloves garlic, finely chopped or minced
1 tbsp ginger, chopped or finely minced
1½ tbsp Curry Powder (recipe, page 164), or to taste
½ cup boiling water (optional)
salt (optional)
garnish:
   1 tbsp chopped coriander (optional)

You can also serve this dip as a soup if you dilute it with 2 cups of chicken stock.

Method:

1. Wash lentils thoroughly, removing those that float.
2. Add 3 cups of water, turmeric and chopped tomato, and boil mixture for 20-30 minutes until lentils are soft and the consistency thick.
3. Heat oil in frying pan, add cumin seeds, curry leaves, onion, garlic and ginger and sauté until golden. Stir in curry powder and sauté for 3-4 minutes more. If mixture is too thick, add about ½ cup of boiling water. Add this to the cooked lentils and stir well. Add salt if desired.
4. Just before serving garnish with chopped coriander. Serve hot as a dip with accompaniments (see list, page 61).

Microwave: cook lentils on 'high' for 20 minutes, otherwise follow the conventional recipe.

To store: cover and refrigerate for up to two days. Reheat before serving.

Nutrition data per total: 2728 kJ (652 cal), CHO 40 g, Protein 17 g, Fat 47 g.

Preparation time: 1 hour. Cooking equipment: saucepan, frying pan.

Dolmades

Serves: 4-6

2 cups chicken stock
1 cup basmati rice, uncooked
1 chicken breast, skinned and minced or finely chopped
1 pkt preserved vine leaves
½ tsp cardamom, freshly crushed
½ tsp salt or 1 chicken stock cube
2 tsp olive oil and 2 tsp extra
1 lemon and juice of ½ lemon extra
½ small finely chopped onion
garnish: 2 tbsp chopped parsley

Method:

1. Bring chicken stock to the boil, reduce heat and simmer.
2. Wash rice and add to the stock.
3. Add chicken. Simmer gently, with lid on, until liquid is absorbed and rice is tender. Add more liquid (water) if necessary. Remove from heat.
4. Rinse vine leaves carefully to remove preserving liquid. Drain.
5. To rice mixture, add flavourings, 2 tsp oil, grated rind and juice of 1 lemon, onion and parsley.
6. Place approximately 1 tbsp of mixture on each vine leaf. Wrap firmly into parcels and place in a baking dish. Continue until all the vine leaves are used. Make sure dolmades are firmly packed into dish.
7. Pour a little water into the baking dish until it reaches about 1 cm (½ in) up the side of the dish, squeeze juice of ½ lemon over, and sprinkle extra 2 tsp olive oil over.
8. Cover with aluminium foil, and bake for about 1 hour.
9. Cool. Remove to a serving dish and serve garnished with parsley.

Accompaniment: Cucumber and Yoghurt Sauce (recipe, page 158).

To store: cover and refrigerate for up to three days. Do not store in an aluminium container.

Nutrition data per serve (if 4 serves): 634 kJ (151 cal), CHO 15 g, Protein 9 g, Fat 6 g.
Preparation time: 2 hours. Cooking equipment: saucepan, baking dish.
Oven temperature: 160°C (325°F)

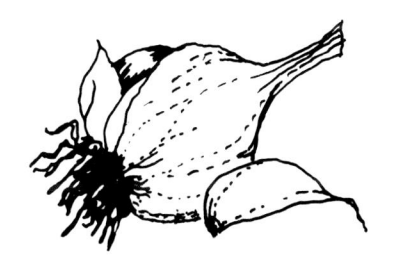

Chick Pea Savoury

Makes: 3 cups

1 cup of dried chick peas
water
2 tsp oil
2 large onions, chopped
2 tsp crushed garlic
2 tsp minced fresh ginger
½ tsp turmeric
1 tsp garam marsala
2 large ripe tomatoes, chopped
2 bay leaves
2 tbsp chopped fresh coriander or mint
lemon juice to taste
salt to taste (optional)

Great served with chappati or flat bread.

Method:

1. Cover the chick peas with water and soak overnight.
2. In a saucepan, heat oil and sauté onion, garlic and ginger until golden, stirring frequently. Add turmeric, garam marsala, tomatoes, bay leaves and half of fresh herbs. Add chick peas and soaking liquid, cover and simmer on low heat until peas are tender. Set aside 1 tbsp of cooked chick peas for the garnish.
3. Remove bay leaves. Blend cooked chick peas in food processor or blender until smooth. Add lemon juice and salt if desired.
4. Sprinkle with remaining fresh herbs and the reserved tablespoon of unpuréed chick peas.

Nutrition data per portion: 3158 kJ (755 cal), CHO 72 g, Protein 28 g, Fat 39 g.

Preparation time: 1½ hours plus overnight. Cooking equipment: saucepan, food processor or blender.

Cheese Puffs

Serves: 4

2 eggs
2 thin slices lean ham, chopped
90 g (3 oz) low-fat block cheese, grated
1 small firm tomato, finely chopped
½ tsp chopped chives
freshly ground black pepper
4 slices of wholemeal bread

Method:

1. Preheat grill.
2. Place eggs in bowl and beat lightly with a fork.
3. Add remaining ingredients, except bread, and mix.
4. Toast bread on one side, remove from the grill and spread the cheese mixture over the untoasted side of the bread.
5. Grill until the mixture puffs up and browns. Serve hot.

Nutrition data per puff: 784 kJ (187 cal), CHO 10 g, Protein 14 g, Fat 10 g.

Preparation time: 15 minutes.

Vegetable Samosas

Serves: 4-8
1-2 per serve

2 medium potatoes, scrubbed and diced
1 medium carrot, scrubbed and diced
½ medium sweet potato, peeled and diced
1 cup frozen peas
1 medium onion, finely chopped
1 tsp olive oil
½ tsp turmeric
2 tsp Curry Powder (recipe, page 164)
½ tsp coriander
½ tsp salt or
  ½ chicken stock cube
1 tsp finely chopped or minced fresh ginger
pepper to taste
200 g (7 oz) low-fat natural yoghurt
12 sheets filo pastry
garnish: sliced cucumber, onion and tomato

Count on serving one or two samosas per person.

Method:

1. Boil, steam or microwave vegetables, except onion, until tender. Cool.
2. Sauté onion in oil till transparent but not brown. Combine with cooked vegetables in a bowl. Add spices. Check flavour and adjust to taste.
3. Using a pastry brush, spread a sheet of filo pastry lightly with yoghurt. Place a second sheet over the first and repeat the procedure. Place a third sheet over this, then cut the pastry in half lengthwise with a sharp knife.
4. Place a generous spoonful of the mixture on one end of the pastry rectangle and fold the filo diagonally to cover the filling. Continue to fold diagonally until all the pastry is folded, making sure that the mixture is totally enclosed.
5. Repeat this procedure until all the pastry is used.
6. Place samosas on a baking sheet. Bake for approximately 15 minutes until brown. Serve with a garnish of sliced cucumber, onion and tomato.

Nutrition data per serve (if 4 serves): 1056 kJ (252 cal), CHO 44 g, Protein 11 g, Fat 4 g.

Preparation time: 1 hour. Cooking equipment: saucepan, frying pan, oven tray. Oven temperature: 180°C (350°F).

Wholemeal Salmon Slices

Serves: 8

440 g (15 oz) can pink salmon
125 g (4 oz) ricotta cheese
juice of 1 lemon
1 tsp curry powder
¼ tsp salt
6 spring onions (shallots), chopped
1 tsp gelatine
2 tbsp hot water
1 wholemeal bread stick

Eat this on the day you make it because it does not keep. Use the soft bread from the centre of the breadstick to make breadcrumbs.

Method:

1. Drain juice from salmon and discard skin and bones.
2. Mash the salmon and mix well with the cheese.
3. Add lemon juice, curry powder, salt and spring onions (shallots).
4. Melt gelatine in hot water, cool slightly, and stir into salmon mixture.
5. Chill in refrigerator for 30 minutes.
6. Cut breadstick into two equal lengths, and remove the crusty ends. Hollow out with knife or spoon. Discard the soft centre.
7. Spoon filling into centres of breadstick and pack in firmly.
8. Wrap in aluminium foil and chill until ready to serve.
9. Slice in 2 cm (¾ in) pieces and serve.

Nutrition data per serve: 600 kJ (143 cal), CHO 6 g, Protein 15 g, Fat 7 g.
Preparation time: 45 minutes.

Mushroom Starter

Makes: 1 cup

¾ cup finely chopped mushrooms
1 tbsp chopped parsley
1 tsp finely chopped chives
¼ tsp ground oregano or ½ tsp of finely chopped fresh oregano
ground black pepper
¼ cup low-fat natural yoghurt
salt to taste

Method:

1. Mix all ingredients and refrigerate for 3 hours before serving.
2. Serve with cut-up fresh vegetables, breads or biscuits (page 61)

Nutrition data per total: 282 kJ (67 cal), CHO 7 g, Protein 9 g, Fat 1 g.
Preparation time: 10 minutes.

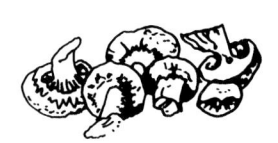

Chinese Dumplings

Makes: 4 serves
4 dumplings per serve

200 g (7 oz) lean minced pork
4 spring onions, (shallots) finely chopped
250 g (8 oz) can bamboo shoots, finely chopped
½ tsp minced ginger
1 tbsp soy sauce
1 egg white
125 g (4 oz) won ton pastry squares
Sauce for dipping:
¼ cup soy sauce with dash of chilli sauce

The won ton pastry squares used in this recipe are available from Asian food stores and some supermarkets.

Method:

1. Combine all ingredients except won ton pastry squares.
2. Place a heaped teaspoonful of mixture onto each won ton pastry square; keep unused pastry covered with a damp tea towel while you are working.
3. Squeeze the pastry up around the filling to make a filled-bag shape.
4. Place dumplings in an oiled steamer and cook over boiling water for approximately 20 minutes.
5. Serve with dipping sauce.

To store: freeze after they are cooked.

Frozen dumplings can be thawed in the microwave. Place them in a covered microwave dish with 2 tbsp water.

Nutrition data per serve : 758 kJ (181 cal), CHO 23 g, Protein 17 g, Fat 2 g.
Preparation time: 45 minutes. Cooking equipment: steamer, saucepan.

Chicken Spread

Makes: 1 cup

1 cup chopped cooked chicken
½ cup almonds or walnuts, chopped
juice of ½ lemon
3 tbsp low-fat natural yoghurt
pinch mustard powder
1 tbsp chopped onion
1 tbsp chopped parsley

Method:

1. Blend all ingredients and refrigerate until ready to serve.
2. Serve on triangles of wholemeal toast, or roll in lettuce to make parcels.

To store: cover and refrigerate up to two days.

Nutrition data per total: 3185 kJ (761 cal), CHO 8 g, Protein 68 g, Fat 51 g.
Preparation time: 15 minutes. Cooking equipment: blender or food processor.

Soups

Minestrone

Serves: 4-6

2 medium onions
2 medium carrots
2 sticks celery
½ capsicum (bell pepper)
2 medium potatoes
125 g (4 oz) green beans, sliced
1 cup shredded cabbage,
4 large tomatoes
2 tsp olive oil
1 cup dried haricot or cannelloni beans
4 cups water
3 bay leaves
½ tsp salt
¼ tsp pepper
juice of ½ lemon
1 tsp dried mixed herbs or 2 tsp fresh mixed herbs

There are dozens of versions of this soup. This one has all the key ingredients of the classic version. To make this soup into a meal-in-one, you can add two cups of cooked wholemeal macaroni just before serving. This provides even more carbohydrate.

Method:

1. Peel and chop vegetables.
2. Heat oil in saucepan.
3. Add onions and cook until lightly browned.
4. Add carrots, celery, capsicum (bell pepper) and potatoes. Cook until lightly coloured.
5. Now add green beans, cabbage and tomatoes. Cook until just tender.
6. Add dried beans, water, herbs and lemon juice.
7. Simmer with lid on until beans are tender (approximately 1 hour).
8. Check for flavour and adjust to taste.
9. Serve with wholemeal breadstick.

To store: cover and refrigerate for up to three days.

Nutrition data per serve: 1105 kJ (264 cal), CHO 40 g, Protein 17 g, Fat 4 g.
Preparation time: 2 hours. Cooking equipment: large saucepan or stock pot.

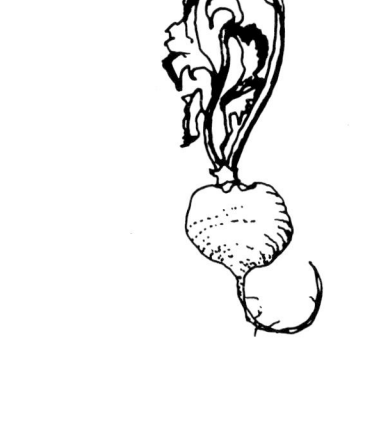

Chicken Stock

Makes: 4 cups

2 medium onions, peeled
1 large carrot
2 sticks celery
1 x 1.5 kg (3 lb) boiling fowl
8 peppercorns
2 bay leaves
sprig of fresh or ¼ tsp dried thyme
5 sprigs parsley
6 cups water
salt to taste

We've given storage options at the end of this recipe because chicken stock is so useful to have on hand. We use it in many other recipes, and it is superior to soup cubes or packet soups.

Method:

1. Wash and roughly chop the vegetables.
2. Place all the ingredients in a large saucepan.
3. Over medium heat, slowly bring mixture to the boil. Skim off any scum that rises to the surface. Reduce heat, cover saucepan, and simmer gently for 3 hours.
4. Strain the soup through a sieve. Reserve the meat for another dish. Discard skin, bones and vegetables.
5. Chill in refrigerator overnight and then skim off any congealed fat. Use in recipes requiring chicken stock or reheat and serve in cups as a nutritious hot beverage.

Nutrition data per serve: negligible.

Preparation time: about 3 hours. Cooking equipment: large saucepan.

To vary: Chicken Soup with Noodles or Rice — just before serving, add half a cup of cooked vermicelli or boiled rice to the hot soup.

To store stock: keep in a sealed container in refrigerator. Clarified stock will keep for a week or two if re-boiled every few days. Freeze in an ice cube tray. Store cubes in a freezer bag for convenience.

Green Pea, Spinach and Chicken Soup

Serves: 4

2 cups frozen peas
3 cups Chicken Stock (see recipe above)
250 g (8 oz) pkt frozen spinach
1 cup chopped, cooked chicken
2 tsp curry powder

Method:

1. Cook peas in stock until tender (approximately 15 minutes).
2. Combine in food processor until partly broken down and return to saucepan.
3. Add spinach and simmer until the spinach is thoroughly heated (approximately 10 minutes).
4. Add chicken and curry powder; bring to the boil and serve.

To store: cover and refrigerate for up to three days.

Nutrition data per serve: 537 kJ (128 cal), CHO 5 g, Protein 20 g, Fat 3 g.

Preparation time: 45 minutes. Cooking equipment: saucepan, food processor or blender.

Eat & Enjoy   Soups

Corn Chowder

Serves: 4

2 tsp margarine
1 large onion, peeled and chopped
2 medium potatoes, peeled
1 chicken stock cube
pinch mixed dried herbs or ½ tsp fresh mixed herbs
pepper to taste
440 g (15 oz) can corn kernels
½ cup water
1½ cups skim or low-fat milk
4 tsp cornflour (cornstarch)

Method:

1. Melt margarine in saucepan. Add onion and cook over low heat until translucent.
2. Cut potatoes into small dice (about 1 cm [½ in] cubes) and add to onion in saucepan.
3. Add stock cube and herbs, pepper, corn and its liquid and the water.
4. Cover and simmer until potatoes are tender (approximately 15 minutes). Now add milk.
5. In a small bowl, blend cornflour (cornstarch) with a little water to a smooth paste. Add to the soup.
6. Bring to the boil, then simmer until slightly thickened, stirring from time to time.
7. Sprinkle with parsley and serve.

Nutrition data per serve: 1032 kJ (246 cal), CHO 44 g, Protein 8 g, Fat 4 g.

Preparation time: 45 minutes. Cooking equipment: large saucepan.

Chinese Chicken and Sweetcorn Soup

Serves: 4

2 tsp peanut oil
2 chicken fillets, finely sliced
2 cloves garlic, crushed
1 tsp chopped ginger
1 litre (1 quart) Chicken Stock (see page 71)
425 g (15 oz) can creamed sweetcorn
1 egg, lightly beaten
garnish: 3 spring onions (shallots)

Method:

1. Place oil in saucepan and heat until moderately hot.
2. Now lightly brown sliced chicken, garlic and ginger. Don't overcook.
3. Add stock and bring to boil.
4. Add creamed corn and simmer for 10 minutes.
5. Remove from heat when ready to serve, then quickly stir in egg to make long strands.
6. Garnish with chopped spring onions (shallots).

To store: cover and refrigerate for up to three days.

Nutrition data per serve: 1029 kJ (246 cal), CHO 26 g, Protein 17 g, Fat 8 g.

Preparation time: 45 minutes. Cooking equipment: saucepan.

Foreground left: Harlequin Salad, right Fettuccine Salmon Salad with Fruity Rice Salad behind it. At the back, filled pita bread.

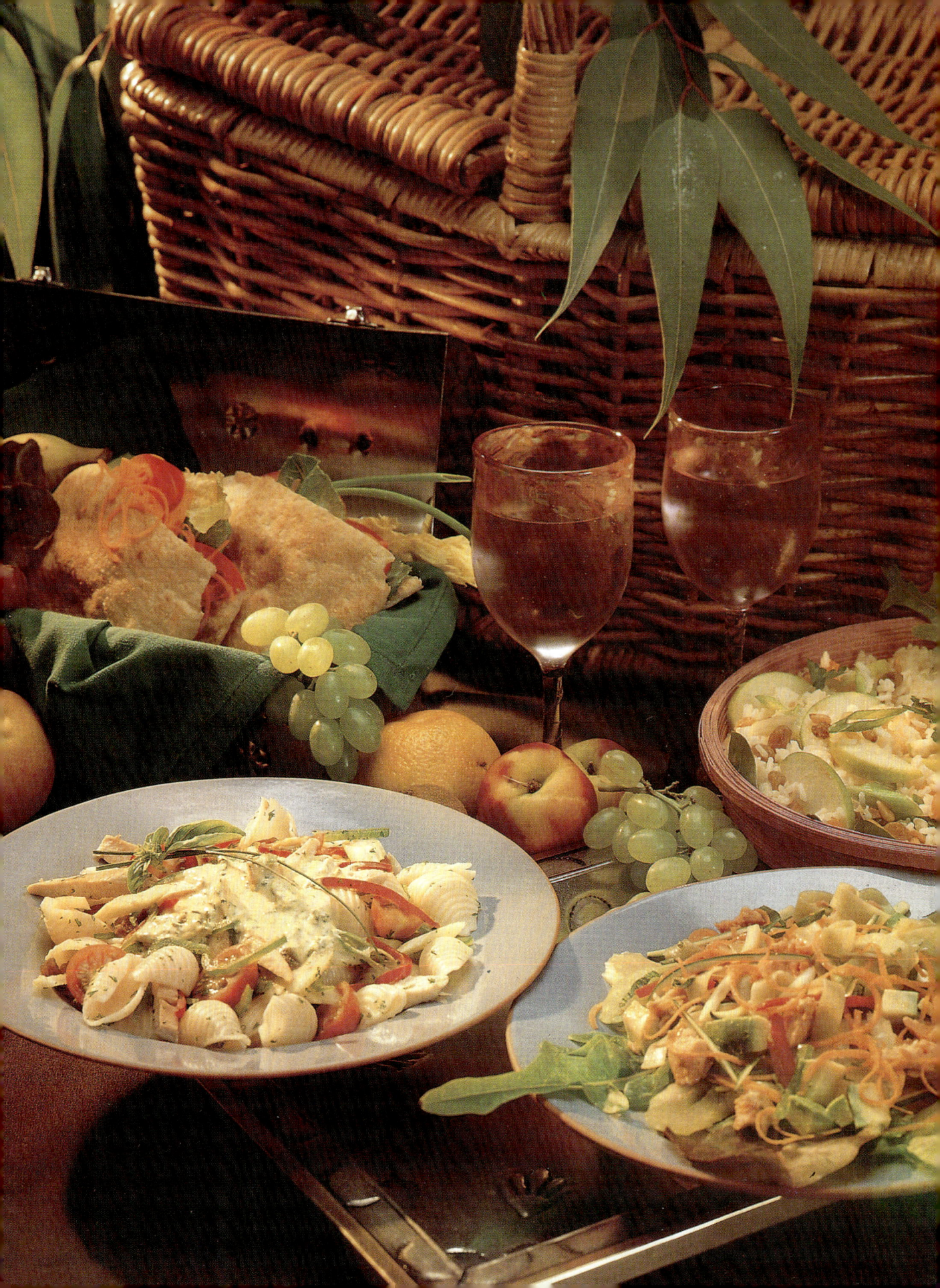

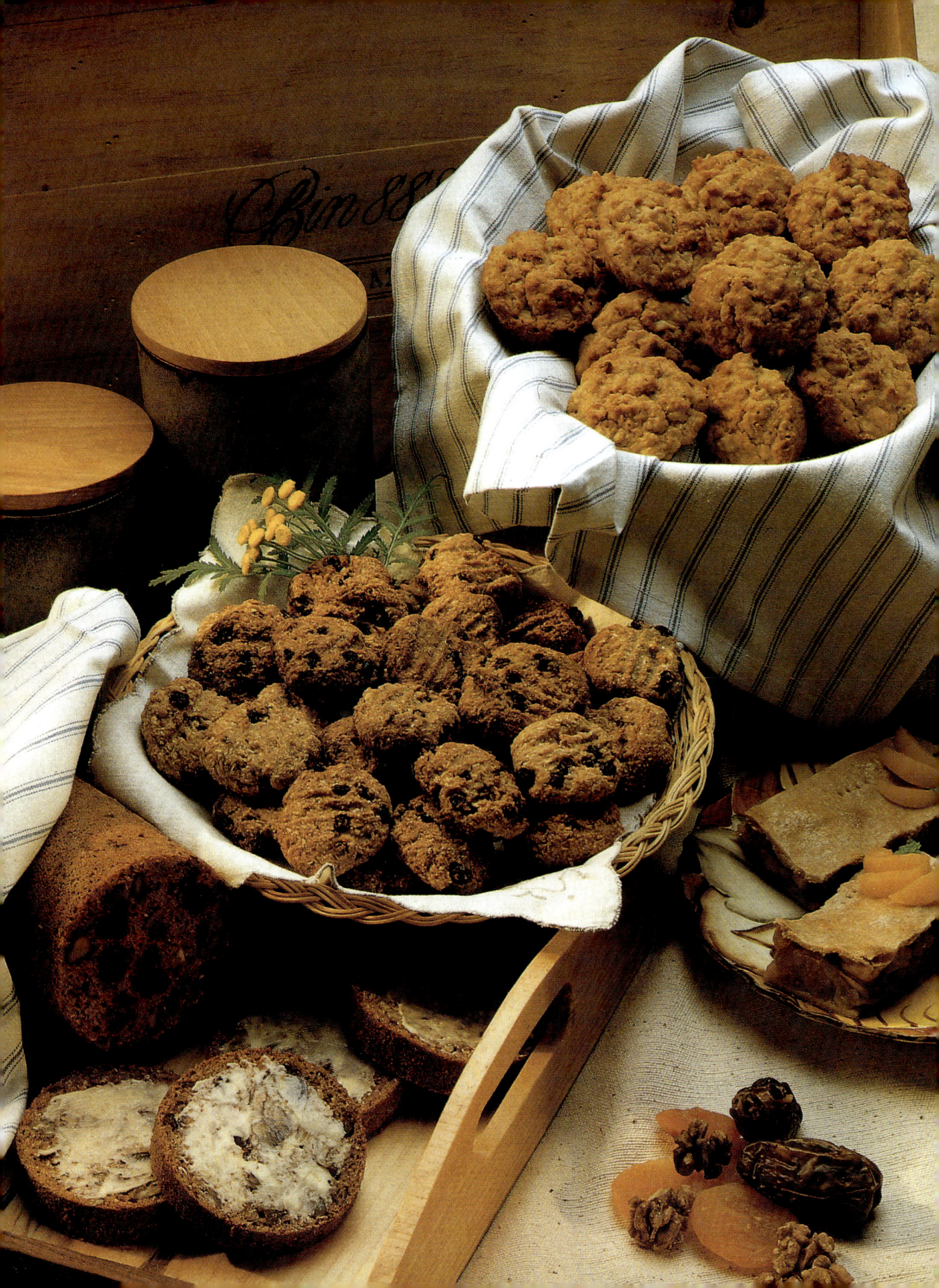

Hot and Sour Soup

Serves: 4

3 chicken fillets
2½ tbsp white vinegar
2 tsp oil
125 g (4 oz) firm tofu (soybean curd) cut into small cubes
4 cups Chicken Stock (see recipe, page 71)
½ medium red capsicum (bell pepper) cut into thin strips
125 g (4 oz) button mushrooms
125 g (4 oz) can bamboo shoots, drained
4 spring onions (shallots), chopped
2 tbsp cornflour (cornstarch)
1 egg
garnish: soy sauce

Method:

1. With a sharp knife, slice chicken very finely.
2. Place chicken slices in bowl with vinegar.
3. Place oil in heavy saucepan and heat on high. Add tofu and stir-fry until tender (about 3 minutes). Remove from saucepan.
4. Pour chicken stock into saucepan with capsicum (bell peppers), mushrooms, bamboo shoots and spring onions (shallots). Heat to boiling, cover and simmer 10 minutes or until vegetables are tender.
5. Add chicken and tofu, heat to boiling.
6. Mix cornflour (cornstarch) and a small amount of water .
7. Slowly stir cornflour (cornstarch) mixture into boiling soup.
8. Cook, stirring constantly, until slightly thickened. Remove from heat.
9. Beat egg in a small bowl.
10. Then slowly pour egg mixture into soup, stirring quickly until egg swirls and has just set.
11. Spoon soup into individual bowls.
12. To each bowl add a dash of soy sauce.

To store: cover and refrigerate for up to three days.

Nutrition data per serve: 1328 kJ (317 cal), CHO 8 g, Protein 28 g, Fat 19 g.

Preparation time: 30 minutes. Cooking equipment: large saucepan.

Foreground: buttered Date and Walnut Loaf, centre right Apple and Apricot Slice with a basket of Chris's Cookies beside it. Banana Muffins at the top.

Singapore Noodle Soup

Serves: 4

300 g (10 oz) green prawns
3 cups water
2 cups chicken stock
180 g (6 oz) barbecued pork, lean
2 tsp sesame oil
2 cloves garlic, finely chopped
½ tsp ginger, finely chopped
100 g (3 oz) fine egg noodles
1 cup bean sprouts, washed and drained
12 spinach leaves, washed and drained
½ tsp five spice powder
garnish:
  110 g (3¼ oz) can crab meat
  4 spring onions (shallots), finely chopped
  ¼ cup cucumber, finely diced

Method:

1. Shell and devein prawns. Wash shells and heads well and shake dry.
2. Bring water to boil, add shells and heads, cover and boil for 20 minutes. Strain.
3. Combine prawn and chicken stocks.
4. Cut pork into thin strips.
5. Heat oil and gently fry garlic and ginger until starting to brown.
6. Add stock and prawns and simmer for 3 minutes.
7. Add noodles and simmer for a further 5 minutes.
8. Add pork, bean sprouts, spinach and five spice powder and simmer for 2 minutes.
9. Pour into a large bowl and garnish with crab meat, spring onions (shallots) and cucumber.

Although a soup this dish makes an ideal light meal.

Nutrition data per serve: 1397 kJ (334 cal), CHO 19 g, Protein 34 g, Fat 13 g.

Preparation time: 45 minutes. Cooking equipment: 1 large saucepan with lid.

Hungarian Soup

Serves: 4

3 cups chicken stock
1 cup finely shredded red cabbage or ¾ cup canned red cabbage, drained
3 small onions, thinly sliced
1 clove garlic, crushed
2 large tomatoes, peeled and quartered
1 large apple, peeled and chopped
coarsely ground black pepper, to taste
¼ tsp ground all spice
garnish: chives

This is a simple, filling and aromatic soup with just a hint of sweetness, ideal for cold winter nights. Eaten with wholemeal bread, it makes a warming supper. For the stock, either use good quality cubes or make your own according to our recipe on page 71.

Method:

1. Place stock in a large saucepan and bring to the boil.
2. Add all other ingredients.
3. Cover and simmer for 30 minutes.
4. Serve, garnished with a sprinkling of chopped chives.

To store: cover and refrigerate for up to three days.

Nutrition data per serve: 213 kJ (51 cal), CHO 10 g, Protein 2 g, Fat trace.

Preparation time: 45 minutes. Cooking equipment: saucepan.

Broccoli and Sweetcorn Soup

Serves: 4

1 large head broccoli
2 cups Chicken Stock (see recipe, page 71)
440 g (15 oz) can creamed sweetcorn
1 stick celery, finely chopped
6 spring onions (shallots), finely sliced
½ tsp salt (optional)
pepper to taste
garnish: chopped chives

Note the high proportion of complex carbohydrate in this delicious soup. Use Chicken Stock recipe on page 71 for a superior result.

Method:

1. Break the broccoli into florets and cook it in stock until tender (approximately 10 minutes).
2. Blend until smooth in food processor.
3. Add creamed sweetcorn, celery, spring onions (shallots) and seasonings.
4. Reheat and serve, garnished with chopped chives.

To store: cover and refrigerate for up to three days.

Nutrition data per serve: 760 kJ (182 cal), CHO 30 g, Protein 9 g, Fat 3 g.

Preparation time: 30 minutes. Cooking equipment: saucepan, food processor or blender.

Curried Carrot and Rice Soup

Serves: 4

4 medium raw carrots, washed and chopped
1 onion, chopped
2 cups water
½ cup raw brown or basmati rice
1 cup water
2 tbsp finely chopped parsley
1 tsp curry powder
½ tsp salt
½ tsp black pepper
1 ½ cups skim milk
garnish: paprika

Although we advocate as little salt as possible in our cooking, it seems to bring out the taste of all the other ingredients in curries.

Method:

1. Cook carrots and onions in 2 cups water until tender. Set aside in its cooking liquid.
2. In the second saucepan, cook rice in 1 cup water until tender (approximately 20-25 minutes). Drain and discard the cooking liquid.
3. Combine carrots, onions and cooking liquid in food processor or blender until smooth.
4. Add to parsley, curry powder, salt, pepper, cooked rice and milk.
5. Return to saucepan and heat until just starting to boil.
6. Remove from the heat and serve, garnished with paprika.

Nutrition data per serve: 668 kJ (160 cal), CHO 31 g, Protein 7 g, Fat 1 g.

Preparation time: 1 hour. Cooking equipment: 2 saucepans, food processor or blender.

Pork and Vegetable Noodle Soup

Serves: 4

200 g (7 oz) bacon bones
4 cups water
250 g (8 oz) pork fillet, diced
1 medium carrot, grated
2 sticks celery, chopped
½ parsnip, grated
½ turnip, grated
1 medium leek, chopped
2 tbsp chopped parsley
½ tsp black pepper
85 g (3 oz) pkt instant noodles
garnish: spring onions (shallots), chopped

The noodles add complex carbohydrate to this nutritious soup.

Method:

1. Place bacon bones and water in saucepan and bring to boil. Simmer for 1 hour. Strain stock and discard the bones.
2. Heat saucepan and dry fry pork fillet until browned.
3. Add pork, carrot, celery, parsnip, turnip, leek, parsley and black pepper to stock.
4. Cook until meat and vegetables are tender.
5. Add noodles and cook a further 5-10 minutes or until noodles are tender, too.
6. Spoon into individual bowls, garnish with chopped spring onions (shallots).

Nutrition data per serve: 633 kJ (151 cal), CHO 16 g, Protein 18 g, Fat 2 g.

Preparation time: 2 hours. Cooking equipment: 2 saucepans.

Beef and Bean Soup

Serves: 4

250 g (8 oz) lean minced beef
1 medium onion, diced
1 small clove garlic
2 sticks celery, diced
410 g (14 oz) can tomatoes
1 tbsp tomato paste
3 cups water
½ tsp oregano, dried, or 1 tsp fresh
½ tsp paprika
½ tsp ground cumin
2 tsp white vinegar
440 g (15 oz) can kidney beans, drained

This hearty soup only needs plenty of wholemeal bread to make it into a meal-in-one.

Method:

1. Dry fry meat, add onion and garlic and cook until juices evaporate and beef is well browned.
2. Add celery, tomatoes, tomato paste, water, oregano, paprika, cumin and vinegar.
3. Bring to boil. Add beans and reduce heat to low, cover and simmer 30 minutes.

To store: cover and refrigerate for up to three days.

Nutrition data per serve: 844 kJ (202 cal), CHO 17 g, Protein 26 g, Fat 3 g.

Preparation time: 1 hour. Cooking equipment: saucepan.

Souper Douper Pumpkin Soup

Serves 4

750 g (1½ lb) pumpkin, peeled, cut into pieces
1 large leek, sliced
3 cups chicken stock
2 tsp mixed dried herbs or 3 tsp fresh herbs
½ tsp coarsely ground black pepper
¼ tsp ground nutmeg
¼ tsp coriander
½ tsp salt
2 tbsp lemon juice
2 tbsp chopped parsley

Method:

1. Place all ingredients except lemon juice and parsley in a saucepan.
2. Bring to the boil and simmer until pumpkin is tender (approximately 20 minutes).
3. Cool slightly, blend in food processor or blender until smooth.
4. Add lemon juice and parsley. Check taste, add salt if needed.
5. Serve with Herby Corn Muffins (see page 188).

To store: cover and refrigerate for up to three days.

Nutrition data per serve: 342 kJ (82 cal), CHO 14 g, Protein 5 g, Fat 1 g.

Preparation time: 1 hour. Cooking equipment: saucepan, food processor or blender.

Gazpacho

Serves: 4

1 small cucumber, peeled
3 spring onions (shallots)
½ red and ½ green capsicum (bell pepper)
2 sticks of celery
4 medium ripe tomatoes or a 425 g (15 oz) can of tomatoes
1 medium white onion
1 cup tomato juice
1 tbsp coarsely ground black pepper
1-2 tsp tabasco sauce, according to taste
garnish: chopped parsley

Method:

1. Finely chop half the cucumber, 3 spring onions (shallots), a quarter of each red and green capsicum (bell pepper), a stick of celery and 1 tomato. Set aside.
2. Roughly chop all remaining vegetables and place in food processor with tomato juice, pepper and tabasco sauce and blend until smooth.
3. Add finely chopped vegetables, mix and chill well.
4. Serve, garnished with chopped parsley.

To store: cover and refrigerate for up to three days.

Nutrition data per serve: 195 kJ (47 cal), CHO 8 g, Protein 3 g, Fat trace.

Preparation time: 25 minutes. Cooking equipment: food processor or blender.

Orange Borscht

Serves: 4

3 cups peeled and grated beetroot
3 cups Chicken Stock (see recipe, page 71)
1 cup unsweetened orange juice
1 cup unsweetened tomato juice
1 sprig fresh thyme or ¼ tsp dried thyme
ground black pepper
garnish: 2 tbsp chopped parsley

Beetroot soup (borscht) is East European in origin and would, traditionally, have been eaten with plain boiled potatoes on the side. You can also add a spoonful of low-fat natural yoghurt to each bowl just before you serve the soup.

Method:

1. Place beetroot and stock in saucepan and bring to the boil. Simmer for 20 minutes.
2. Strain stock into a clean saucepan and add 1 cup of the cooked beetroot. Discard the remaining beetroot.
3. Add the juices, thyme and pepper.
4. Bring to boil and remove sprig of thyme.
5. Serve in bowls and sprinkle with chopped parsley.

To store: cover and refrigerate for up to three days.

Nutrition data per serve: 263 kJ (63 cal), CHO 13 g, Protein 2 g, Fat trace.

Preparation time: 30 minutes. Cooking equipment: 2 large saucepans.

Entrées and Light Meals

Wholemeal Beef and Bean Burritos

Serves: 4

Tortillas:

1 cup each, wholemeal flour and plain flour
2 tsp baking powder
½ tsp salt
1 cup warm water

Filling:

500 g (1 lb) lean minced steak
1 medium onion, chopped
1 beef stock cube or ½ tsp salt
½ tsp pepper
150 g (5 oz) tomato paste
100 mL (3 fl oz) water
tabasco sauce to taste
juice of ½ lemon
410 g (15 oz) can red kidney beans, rinsed and drained
garnish: shredded lettuce and finely chopped onion

Method:

Filling:

1. Dry fry meat until lightly browned. Add onion and continue to sauté until browned.
2. Add crumbled stock cube, pepper, tomato paste, water, tabasco sauce and lemon juice. Stir until well combined. Add kidney beans and mix in well. Bring to the boil, turn down the heat and simmer 10-15 minutes until the meat is cooked.
3. Add extra water if necessary to make a thick sauce.
4. Keep meat and bean mixture warm until tortillas are ready or allow to cool, refrigerate and reheat when needed.

Tortillas:

5. Sift flours, baking powder and salt.
6. Gradually stir in warm water to form a dough.
7. Turn dough onto floured board and knead until smooth. Cover with plastic film and allow to rest 15-20 minutes.
8. Cut into 12 equal pieces. Shape each into a ball.
9. Flatten each ball into a 10-12 cm (4-5 in) patty, roll into a very thin, round pastry, approximately 20-22 cm (9-10 in), making sure dough and rolling pin are well floured to prevent sticking.
10. Heat frying pan. Place each tortilla on dry surface of frying pan. As blisters appear, press gently with egg slice or spatula. When underside is brown, turn over and cook until blisters have formed on other side and tortilla is lightly browned.
11. Lift onto tray covered with a damp tea towel. Fold tea towel to cover tortilla.
12. Repeat until all tortillas are cooked.
13. Place some hot filling onto each tortilla and roll up. Serve immediately. They should be eaten with the fingers.
14. To serve, sprinkle lightly with lettuce and onion if desired.

Nutrition data per serve: *2233 kJ (533 cal), CHO 66 g, Protein 59 g, Fat 7 g.*
Preparation time: 2 hours. Cooking equipment: frying pan.

Prosciutto and Rock Melon (Cantaloupe)

Serves: 4

½ ripe rock melon (cantaloupe), peeled and seeded

12 slices paper-thin lean prosciutto

4 lettuce leaves

Method:

1. Cut melon into two and each half into six pieces, evenly shaped to give 12 pieces.
2. Wrap each piece in a slice of prosciutto and secure with a toothpick.
3. Arrange lettuce leaves on four individual plates and top each with three pieces of melon and prosciutto. Serve chilled.

Nutrition data per serve: 189 kJ (45 cal), CHO 1 g, Protein 5 g, Fat 2 g.

Preparation time: 15 minutes.

To vary: use honey dew melon instead of rock melon if you wish. Try using smoked pork or smoked beef instead of prosciutto.

Harlequin Noodle Salad

Serves: 4

1 cup shell noodles, uncooked

1 cup cooked and diced chicken fillets

½ cup diced celery

1 small green and
1 small red capsicum (bell pepper), chopped

4 spring onions (shallots), chopped

1 tbsp chopped parsley

½ cup sultanas

black pepper to taste

dressing: ½ quantity Curry Dressing (see recipe, page 161)

garnish: 4 lettuce cups

Make this the day before you want to serve it, so the flavour can develop.

Method:

1. Place noodles in saucepan of boiling water. Cook until tender and then drain.
2. Combine cooked noodles, diced chicken, celery, capsicum (bell pepper), spring onions (shallots), parsley, sultanas and black pepper.
3. Mix in the curry dressing.
4. Refrigerate for 1 hour.
5. Serve in lettuce cups.

To store: keep in airtight container in refrigerator for up to two days.

Nutrition data per serve: 950 kJ (227 cal), CHO 34 g, Protein 16 g, Fat 3 g.

Preparation time: 1½ hours plus preparation time for dressing.
Cooking equipment: saucepan.

Spinach Ravioli with Fresh Tomato Sauce

Serves: 4

6 large ripe tomatoes, roughly chopped
1 tsp sugar
1 tsp chopped fresh basil or ½ tsp dried basil
pinch tarragon
375 g (12 oz) fresh spinach ravioli
60 g (2 oz) low-fat block cheese, grated

Method:

1. Place tomatoes, sugar and herbs in saucepan and simmer gently until mixture forms a thick sauce.
2. While tomatoes are cooking, threequarter fill a second saucepan with cold water and rapidly bring to boil. Add ravioli and cook until tender. Drain.
3. Pour sauce over ravioli and mix gently.
4. Sprinkle with cheese.

Nutrition data per serve: 1307 kJ (312 cal), CHO 51 g, Protein 15 g, Fat 5 g.

Preparation time: 45 minutes. Cooking equipment: 2 saucepans.

Bombay Burgers with Cucumber and Yoghurt Sauce

Serves: 4
Makes 12 patties

1 cup dried red lentils
1 large potato, cut into pieces
1 medium onion, finely chopped
¼ cup shredded coconut
1 tbsp sesame seeds
1 tbsp plain flour
1 tsp curry powder
1 tsp finely chopped fresh ginger
½ tsp salt
¼ tsp pepper
2 tsp lemon juice
¾–1 cup wheatgerm or wholegrain breadcrumbs
garnish:
sliced onion rings
1 quantity of Cucumber and Yoghurt Sauce (recipe page 158)

Method:

1. Soak lentils in water for 2 hours.
2. Rinse, cover with water in a saucepan and simmer for approximately 30 minutes until tender. Add potato 10 minutes into the cooking time. Alternatively, place lentils in a bowl with water and microwave on 'high' for 20 minutes or until tender. Add potato 10 minutes into the cooking time.
3. Drain any liquid from lentils and potato, and mash thoroughly. Add onion, coconut, sesame seeds, flour, spices and lemon juice.
4. Allow to cool (preferably chill).
5. Shape into patties and coat with wheatgerm or breadcrumbs.
6. Bake on lightly oiled tray for 10-15 minutes, or cook in a frying pan lightly brushed with oil, taking care not to burn the coating.
7. Serve hot garnished with onion rings and with Cucumber and Yoghurt Sauce.

Nutrition data per serve: 838 kJ (200 cal), CHO 22 g, Protein 10 g, Fat 8 g.

Preparation time: 1 hour plus preparation time for sauce.
Cooking equipment: saucepan, oven tray or frying pan.
Oven temperature: 190°C (375°F).

Crêpes and Pancakes

Serves: 4
Makes: 12 large or 24 small crêpes

Crêpes
1 cup wholemeal or plain white flour or half and half
3 eggs, lightly beaten
2 tsp oil or melted butter
1½ cups skim milk

Crêpes are small, very thin pancakes; the raw batter is thinner than for traditional pancakes.

Pancakes make a large, hearty wrapping for a variety of fillings. The cooked pancake should be about 2 mm (⅛ in) thick.

Both crêpes and pancakes are simple to make and very versatile. With either savoury or sweet fillings, use them for entrées, main courses, desserts or snacks.

You will find that crêpes made entirely with wholemeal flour tend to be heavy. A half-and-half combination makes a nutritious and tasty version.

Method:

1. Using a food processor or blender, add all ingredients at once and process until smooth.
   Working by hand, sift flour into a bowl (if using wholemeal flour, add any wheat husks left in sieve to the sifted flour). Make a well in the flour. Slowly add the beaten eggs, stirring continually to draw the ingredients together and prevent lumps forming. Mix oil or melted butter with milk. Slowly add to flour mixture, stirring continually, to form a thin, smooth pouring consistency like that of thin pouring cream. If too thick, add more milk, a little at a time, until you have the right consistency.
2. Transfer batter to a jug and leave to stand in a cool place for at least an hour. If the mixture has thickened, add more milk, a little at a time, to the consistency of thin pouring cream.
3. Lightly grease a crêpe or heavy-bottomed frying pan and heat until very hot, but not smoking. Pour in 2-4 tbsp of batter, depending on size of pan, tilt pan to spread batter evenly.
4. When fine bubbles appear on the surface of the crêpe and it appears dry, use an egg slice or spatula to flip over and cook the other side for approximately 5 seconds until pale golden brown.

5. Repeat these steps for the remainder of the batter, brushing the pan with a little oil between crêpes and stacking them as they are cooked. Keep them covered with a damp tea towel until you need them.

Use any of the filling mixtures on page 84, or create your own. Crêpes can be filled and then served rolled up or folded in half or in quarters.

To store: you may prepare crêpes and pancakes ahead of time. Cover and refrigerate for up to two days, or pack in freezer bags, with a layer of waxed paper or plastic film between each crêpe, and freeze.

Nutrition data per serve (3 crêpes): 968 kJ (231 cal), CHO 29, Protein 12 g, Fat 7 g.
Preparation time: batter 10 minutes, standing time for raw batter 1 hour, cooking time 20 minutes.
Cooking equipment: jug, crêpe pan or small frying pan.

Serves: 4-5 (makes 8-10 pancakes)

Pancakes

¾ cup wholemeal or plain white flour or half-and-half
1 egg
1¼–1½ cups skim milk

This is a traditional recipe. Pancakes are larger and heavier-textured than crêpes. The pancakes should be about the size of a dinner plate and about 2 mm (⅛ in) thick. The same guidelines we set out at the start of the crêpe recipe apply here.

Method:

Exactly as for crêpes

To store: as for crêpes

Nutrition data per serve (2 pancakes): 778 kJ (186 cal), CHO 26 g, Protein 9 g, Fat 5 g.
Preparation time: batter 10 minutes, standing time for raw batter 1 hour, cooking time 20 minutes.
Cooking equipment: jug, small frying pan.

Savoury Fillings for Crêpes or Pancakes

Allow three crêpes or two pancakes per serve. Fill pancakes with any of the fillings that follow, and top with low-fat natural yoghurt or ricotta cheese or a fine sprinkling of parmesan cheese.

Serve the filled pancakes hot, accompanied by a crisp, green salad.

Ham and asparagus	Diced lean ham and cooked asparagus spears or pieces tossed in Cheese Sauce (recipe, page 155).
Mushroom and onion	Sliced mushrooms and onions cooked in a frying pan brushed with oil and tossed in White Sauce (recipe, page 154).
Ratatouille	Ratatouille Sauce (recipe, page 157) and topped with grated low-fat block cheese.
Spinach	Cooked, chopped spinach mixed with ricotta cheese, sautéed spring onions (shallots), chopped basil and pine nuts.
Seafood	500 g (1 lb) seafood (e.g. marinara mix) cooked in one quantity of Tomato and Basil Sauce (recipe, page 156).
Chicken and avocado	Two sliced cooked chicken fillets and one sliced avocado tossed in one quantity Cheese Sauce (see recipe, page 155).
Savoury beef	500 g (1 lb) lean minced beef cooked in one quantity of Tomato and Basil Sauce (recipe, page 156). Fill crêpes or pancakes and top with low-fat natural yoghurt or ricotta cheese, or a fine sprinkling of parmesan cheese.
Steak and onion	Slice 500 g (1 lb) fillet steak into very thin strips, and marinate in 2 tbsp Worcestershire sauce and 1 crushed clove of garlic for 10 minutes. Sauté beef in 2 tsp oil for 3 minutes. Add 1 large sliced onion and sauté for another 2 minutes. Add ¼ cup red wine, and simmer for 1-2 minutes. Thicken with 1 tbsp cornflour (cornstarch) blended with 2 tbsp water. Fill pancakes and serve them topped with low-fat natural yoghurt and a sprinkling of chopped parsley.
Red kidney bean and corn	Sauté 1 medium finely diced capsicum (bell pepper) and 1 medium finely chopped onion in 3 tbsp water for approximately 3 minutes until soft. Add 1 cup drained canned red kidney beans, 1 cup drained canned corn kernels, 2 tbsp tomato paste, ¼ tsp ground oregano and a small pinch chilli powder. Simmer gently for 5-10 minutes until the liquid is almost evaporated. Fill the pancakes and roll them up. Sprinkle with 4 tbsp low-fat grated cheese, and grill to melt the cheese topping.

Pasties (and Filo Rolls)

Serves: 4

200 g (7 oz) rump, porterhouse or fillet steak
1 potato, finely diced
1 medium carrot, finely diced
1 small turnip, finely diced
1 small onion, finely diced
¼ tsp white pepper
¼ tsp dried mixed herbs
2 tbsp finely chopped parsley
1 quantity Wholemeal Pastry (recipe page 190)
1 tbsp water
2 tbsp skim milk, for glazing

As a main course, serve pasties with vegetables and Tomato and Basil Sauce (recipe, page 156). They also make a wonderful light lunch or meal, served with salad.

Method:

1. Cut meat into small cubes, about 1 cm x 1 cm (½ in x ½ in).
2. In a bowl, combine meat, diced vegetables, pepper and herbs.
3. Divide pastry into four portions. Roll out each portion to about the size of a saucer.
4. Divide the meat mixture between the rounds, placing meat slightly off the centre of each round.
5. Brush the edges of the pastry with a little water. Fold pastry over, in half, to make a pasty shape.
6. Use the back of a fork to crimp the edges of the pasties firmly.
7. Place the finished pasties on a lightly greased baking tray. Prick the top of each pasty three times with a fork. Brush the surface of each pasty with a little skim milk.
8. Bake for 35 minutes or until browned.

To freeze: prepare the pasties to Step 6, place in freezer bags or other suitable container. Defrost before baking, as above.

Nutrition data per serve: 2374 kJ (567 cal), CHO 56 g, Protein 22 g, Fat 28 g.
Preparation time: 1½ hours. Cooking equipment: baking tray. Oven temperature: 200°C (400°F).

Filo Rolls

Makes 4 rolls

This variation of pasties keeps the fat content down — 12 sheets of filo pastry are all you need to make four rolls.

Method

1. Precook the meat and vegetables by combining them in a saucepan with ½ cup of water and simmering them for 10 minutes. Drain.

2. Use 3 sheets of filo pastry per roll, folding each sheet in half to make 6 layers. Brush skim milk between the layers of the filo pastry. Divide the meat mixture into 4 and place a portion on each portion of filo and roll them into parcels. Brush the inner edges of the filo with a little skim milk and press down gently to seal. Glaze the tops of the rolls lightly with skim milk. Bake for 15-20 minutes, or until crisp and lightly brown.

To store: cover and refrigerate for up to two days. Reheat slowly but thoroughly. If you want to freeze them, do so before you bake them. Later thaw and bake them as above.

Nutrition data per serve: 860 kJ (205 cal), CHO 28 g, Protein 16 g, Fat 3 g.

Gado Gado

Serves: 4

1 cup bean shoots
1 cup green beans, string removed
1½ cups broccoli florets
1 cup carrot rings
1 cup cabbage, diced
1 medium green capsicum (bell pepper), sliced
6-10 snow peas
2 tomatoes, cut into wedges
2 onions, cut into wedges
1 small cucumber, peeled and diced
2 hard-boiled eggs, cut into quarters

You have free rein with this recipe to add or change vegetables according to season or taste.

Method:

1. Half fill a medium saucepan with water and bring to a rapid boil. Plunge the vegetables, except the tomatoes and cucumber, one variety at a time, into the boiling water for no more than 1 minute, or until the colour intensifies, or microwave with 2 tbsp water on 'high' for 2 minutes. Quickly remove the blanched vegetables from the water, place in the colander and immediately flush with cold, running water; this preserves the colour and crispness. Bring water back to the boil before blanching each type of vegetable.
2. Arrange all the ingredients on a platter.
3. Serve as an appetizer or entrée at either room temperature or chilled with cooked brown rice and a dish of warm Saté (Peanut) Sauce (recipe, page 155).

To store: cover and refrigerate for no more than one day.

Nutrition data per serve: 433 kJ (103 cal), CHO 10 g, Protein 9 g, Fat 3 g.

Preparation time: 30 minutes. Cooking equipment: medium saucepan, large saucepan.

Fish and Seafood

The beauty of fish and seafood is that they have plenty of protein, vitamins and minerals and little fat. This gives them a kilojoule/energy value less than an equivalent serve of meat and makes fish and seafood an invaluable, and delicious, part of your regular meal plan.

Cooking fish and seafood

Baking

Whole fish (large or small), cutlets or fish fillets are all equally good cooked this way. Place the fish in a shallow casserole and flavour it to taste, for instance with a sliced onion, a bay leaf, herbs of your choice and a few peppercorns, a little salt (optional). Then pour over the fish approximately 1/2-1 cup of liquid depending on the amount of fish. The liquid can be low-fat milk, wine or tomato juice. Bake, covered, at 180°C (350°F) for 15-20 minutes or until the fish flakes when you test it with a fork.

Alternatively, place the fish on foil, sprinkle with lemon juice and herbs, seal, and then cook as above without any additional liquid.

Grilling

Allow 5-8 minutes for fillets, cutlets, kebabs or small fish; 10 minutes for medium-sized whole fish and 15-20 minutes for large whole fish. Watch the fish carefully while it grills, turning it once or twice, or it will overcook and dry out.

We have given some lovely marinade recipes in this book which you can use to flavour the fish before and use as a baste while cooking. Grilled fish is delicious cooked with no more than a sprinkling of herbs, lemon juice, black pepper and a little salt (optional).

Poaching

With this method the fish cooks in a flavoured, simmering liquid. Place the fish in a shallow saucepan with a lid, add just enough liquid (milk, stock or wine or a combination of any two of these) to barely cover the fish and then season it to taste. You can, for instance, add sliced onion, bay leaf, peppercorns, ground black pepper, parsley and a sliced carrot which will give you a wonderfully flavoursome result. Add salt if you like.

Cover and simmer gently on the stove for 5-8 minutes if you are using thin fillets, or for about 10 minutes if you are using thicker pieces. Again, use the test of flaking the fish with a fork to check when it's ready and take it off the heat immediately. Use the poaching liquid as the base for sauce.

Microwaving

Fish and seafood are excellent cooked in the microwave. Place fish in the microwave dish, add 1/4 cup of liquid such as wine, stock or low-fat milk, flavour as for poaching or baking above, cover with plastic wrap and cook the fish on 'high'. Allow 3 minutes for small fillets, 5-7 minutes for larger fillets or small whole fish and 10-12 minutes for large whole fish. Arrange the seafood in a single layer in a shallow dish. Cover with plastic wrap and cook on 'medium' until opaque (approximately 3-4 minutes). Stand, covered, for 5 minutes before serving.

Fish with Various Sauces

Grill 4 fillets of white fish such as snapper, flathead, whiting, sea perch on both sides until cooked through (approximately 8-10 minutes). Alternatively, cover and microwave on 'medium-high' for 4-6 minutes. Serve topped with a sauce such as:

Green Champagne (recipe, page 159)   **Black Bean (recipe, page 157)**

Ratatouille (recipe, page 157)   **Sweet and Sour (recipe, page 159)**

Curried Tuna and Rice Casserole

Serves: 4

425 g (15 oz) tuna canned in brine
juice of 1 lemon
120 g (4 oz) raw brown rice
Sauce:
2 small onions, diced
3 tsp curry powder
2 tbsp wholemeal flour
3 cups skim milk
2 slices wholemeal bread, crumbed

Replace tuna with salmon if you prefer.

Method:

1. Mix tuna and lemon juice in bowl.
2. Cook brown rice in boiling water.
3. Drain rice and combine with the tuna mixture.
4. Dry fry onion and curry powder in a saucepan.
5. Combine flour with a little milk to make a smooth paste.
6. Add remaining milk to onions and curry powder and bring to the boil. Remove from heat and add the flour paste.
7. Return to heat and stir continually until mixture thickens.
8. Pour two-thirds of the curry sauce over tuna and rice. Mix.
9. Spoon into a casserole, pour the remaining sauce over the top.
10. Cover with breadcrumbs, and bake in the oven until golden and the casserole is heated through (approximately 30 minutes).

To store: cover and refrigerate for 24 hours.

Nutrition data per serve: 1527 kJ (365 cal), CHO 45 g, Protein 36 g, Fat 4 g.
Preparation time: 1 hour 40 minutes. Cooking equipment: 2 saucepans, casserole.
Oven temperature: 160°C (325°F).

Piquant Fish in Foil

Serves: 4

4 large fillets of fish (e.g. sea perch or barracouta), or small whole fish (e.g. whiting or bream)
2 tsp finely chopped, fresh tarragon or
½ tsp dried
1 tbsp very finely chopped parsley (optional)
coarsely ground black pepper, to taste
1 medium onion, thinly sliced
1 lemon, thinly sliced
juice of 1 lemon
2 tbsp dry white wine (optional)

This is a wonderful way to prepare fresh fish. Serve it with jacket potatoes and a crisp salad.

Method:

1. Use four pieces of foil large enough to completely wrap the fish fillets. Lightly grease the foil or spray it well with non-stick cooking spray.
2. Place the fish fillets on the pieces of foil. Sprinkle each fillet with the herbs and black pepper. Arrange several onion rings on top of each fillet and top with one or two slices of lemon.
3. Mix lemon juice and white wine and pour over the fish.
4. Wrap each fillet in foil, sealing along the top, so that the juices aren't lost during cooking or when opening the foil.
5. Place the foil parcels, sealed side up, on a baking tray. Bake or barbecue for 30 minutes.
6. Open foil along the sealing edge and serve immediately.

Nutrition data per serve: 623 kJ (149 cal), CHO 2 g, Protein 27 g, Fat 3 g.

Preparation time: 30-40 minutes. Cooking equipment: baking tray. Oven temperature: 180°C (350°F). Barbecue: glowing coals.

Fish in Orange Sauce

Serves: 4

juice of 2 oranges
juice of 1 lemon
1 tsp margarine
¼ tsp black pepper, coarsely ground
4 fillets fish
small quantity of plain flour

Method:

1. Place juices, margarine and pepper in pan.
2. Cook until slightly reduced.
3. Dust fish with flour.
4. Add to sauce and poach until just cooked, turning once.
5. Lift out onto serving plates. Spoon sauce over.

Nutrition data per serve: 693 kJ (166 cal), CHO 4 g, Protein 27 g, Fat 4 g.

Preparation time: 15 minutes. Cooking equipment: frying pan.

Eat & Enjoy   *Fish and Seafood*   89

Seafood Pasta

Serves: 4

300 g (10 oz) pasta (spaghetti, tagliatelle or macaroni), uncooked
2 tbsp water
½ medium onion, chopped
1 clove garlic, crushed
1 cup skim milk
2 tsp cornflour (cornstarch)
1½ cups mixed cooked seafood (oysters, calamari, shrimps, clams, scallops)
1 tbsp parsley, chopped
coarsely ground black pepper to taste
salt to taste

Method:

1. Fill a large saucepan to two-thirds with water, and bring to a rapid boil. Add pasta, and boil rapidly for 10-12 minutes until *al dente* (tender, but still firm to bite).
2. While the pasta is cooking, prepare the sauce. In a medium saucepan, boil the 2 tbsp of water. Add the onion and garlic and cook until tender.
3. In a small bowl, blend 1 tbsp of the milk with the cornflour (cornstarch) to make a smooth paste. Then stir in the remainder of the milk. Add mixture to the onion and garlic, and stir constantly over medium heat until sauce thickens.
4. Over medium heat, add all the remaining ingredients, and stir to combine and heat through.
5. Drain the pasta and add to the sauce. Toss gently to combine.
6. Serve at once.

Nutrition data per serve: 1495 kJ (357 cal), CHO 48 g, Protein 31 g, Fat 4 g.

Preparation time: 30 minutes. Cooking equipment: large saucepan, medium saucepan.

Whole Fish in Ginger

Serves: 4

1 kg whole fish (e.g. snapper, blue eye or coral trout), gutted and scaled, but with head intact
2 tsp chopped ginger
1 clove garlic, crushed
¼ cup soy sauce
juice of 1 lemon

Method:

1. Using a very sharp knife, score the skin of the fish on each side, three or four times, at equal intervals and at an angle to the backbone.
2. Place fish on its side in a flat dish, or support it upright with wooden skewers.
3. Combine remaining ingredients to make a marinade, and pour over the fish.
4. Bake the fish, uncovered, for 30 minutes or until fish flakes when tested with a fork. Baste frequently with the marinade during cooking.

¾ cup dry white wine
4 spring onions, sliced lengthways
garnish: thin slices of lemon

5. Serve the fish whole with cooking juices and garnished with lemon slices. Accompany with boiled brown rice and a green salad.

Microwave method:

At step 4, cover with plastic film and cook on 'high' for 15 minutes.

Nutrition data per serve: 497 kJ (119 cal), CHO 1 g, Protein 22 g, Fat 3 g.
Preparation time: 40 minutes. Cooking equipment: shallow casserole.
Oven temperature: 180°C (350°F).

Vegetable-stuffed Trout

Serves: 4

4 small trout, ready to cook
juice of 2 lemons
2 tbsp mixed fresh herbs, chopped (e.g. thyme, parsley, marjoram)
4 spring onions (shallots), finely chopped
1 tbsp finely chopped celery
2 tbsp finely chopped green capsicum (bell pepper)
4 mushrooms, finely chopped
1 tsp ground black pepper

Serve the trout with plenty of noodles, rice or potatoes, plus a salad, and you have a well-rounded main course.

Method:

1. Wash fish.
2. Place each fish on a piece of aluminium foil large enough to wrap it up completely.
3. Pour lemon juice over the outside and inside of fish.
4. Combine all other ingredients in a mixing bowl.
5. Divide into four and pack a quarter of the mixture into the cavity of each fish.
6. Wrap firmly in foil. Seal edges carefully.
7. Bake in oven or under grill until cooked through (approximately 10-15 minutes).

Microwave method:

Follow the same method as above except use a suitable large shallow microwave dish, and secure the cavity of each fish with toothpicks. Cover dish with plastic film. Bake on 'medium-high' for 8-12 minutes. Let stand, covered, for 5 minutes before serving.

Nutrition data per serve: 511 kJ (122 cal), CHO 1 g, Protein 23 g, Fat 3 g.
Preparation time: 20 minutes.
Cooking equipment: baking dish. Oven temperature: 180°C (350°F), or use griller.

Pasta and Smoked Trout

Serves: 4

250 g (8 oz) uncooked fettucine
1 medium smoked trout
½ cup dry white wine
½ tsp granulated garlic (or 1 clove, chopped)
½ tsp dry mustard
½ quantity White Sauce (recipe, page 154)
garnish: 1 tbsp chopped capers

Method:

1. Boil fettucine in water as directed on the pack, and drain.
2. While pasta is cooking, skin the trout and remove the flesh from the bones by lifting it off with a fork. Break the flesh into bite size pieces.
3. Mix wine, garlic and mustard, and bring to the boil in large saucepan. Add the white sauce and gently reheat.
4. Add the fettucine and mix through, reheating gently.
5. Add the fish, mixing carefully. When the fish is hot, turn it onto a serving dish and sprinkle with capers.

Nutrition data per serve: 1490 kJ (356 cal), CHO 48 g, Protein 28 g, Fat 5 g.

Preparation time: 30-35 minutes, including time for preparing white sauce.
Cooking equipment: 2 large saucepans.

Crab and Zucchini Quiche

Serves: 4

1 quantity Wholemeal Pastry (recipe, page 190)
170 g (6 oz) can crab meat
1 zucchini, sliced
2 spring onions (shallots), chopped
¼ cup ricotta cheese
4 eggs
1 cup skim milk
1 cup low-fat natural yoghurt
pepper to taste
¼ tsp salt (optional)

You can make it just as successfully with shrimps in place of the crab, or using fresh seafood instead of canned. Asparagus or mushrooms make a delicious substitute for the zucchini.

Method:

1. Roll out pastry and line flan dish.
2. Place crab meat, sliced zucchini and spring onions (shallots) over base of pastry.
3. Blend all other ingredients and pour over filling.
4. Bake 30-45 minutes or until filling is set.

To store: cover and refrigerate for up to 2 days. Do not reheat or the filling will toughen.

Nutrition data per serve: 2737 kJ (654 cal), CHO 56 g, Protein 30 g, Fat 34 g.

Preparation time: 45-60 minutes. Cooking equipment: flan dish.
Oven temperature: 180°C (350°F).

No. 4

Paella

Serves: 8

2 tsp olive oil
8 small chicken pieces (no wings), skin removed
pinch salt and black pepper
1 large onion, chopped
2 large tomatoes, chopped
1 tsp chopped, crushed or minced garlic
¼ tsp saffron powder
2 cups uncooked, long grain brown, or basmati rice
2 cups water
1 chicken stock cube
1 small green or red capsicum (bell pepper), cut into strips
1 cup frozen peas
12 cooked king prawns, heads removed, shelled and cleaned (tails left on)

This is a wonderful dinner party or luncheon dish served with a green salad and crusty wholemeal bread.

Method:

1. Heat oil in frying pan.
2. Sprinkle chicken pieces lightly with black pepper and a pinch of salt (if desired).
3. Add to frying pan and brown well on all sides. Remove from the frying pan and set aside on a plate.
4. Add onion to pan and brown.
5. Add tomato and garlic, cook until soft.
6. Add saffron and rice. Stir.
7. Pour in water and stock cube, and mix well.
8. Spoon into casserole.
9. Stir capsicum (bell pepper) strips, peas and chicken pieces into mixture.
10. Cover and cook in a preheated oven until rice is cooked through and liquid absorbed (approximately 1-2 hours).
11. Just before serving, add the prawns and allow to heat through. Serve immediately from the casserole.

Nutrition data per serve: 1312 kJ (313 cal), CHO 41 g, Protein 24 g, Fat 5 g.

Preparation time: 2-3 hours. Cooking equipment: frying pan, large shallow casserole. Oven temperature: 200°C (400°F).

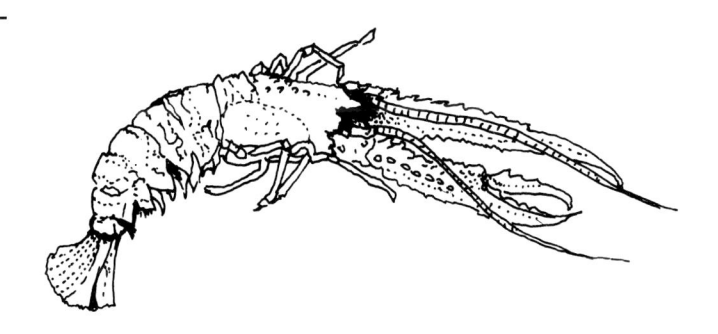

Mussels à la Grecque

Serves: 4

2 tsp olive oil
2 medium leeks, sliced
3 large peeled tomatoes or 425 g (15 oz) can tomatoes, chopped
1 tbsp tomato paste
¼ tsp ground basil
½ tsp ground oregano
ground black pepper to taste
salt to taste (not needed if you use canned tomatoes)
1½ kg (3 lb) mussels in shells, scrubbed and beards removed

Black mussels are ideal for this recipe. However, it's also excellent with clams or pipis. Green-lipped mussels are also perfect for cooking this way.

Method:

1. Heat oil in a saucepan and sauté leeks until tender.
2. Add tomatoes, tomato paste, basil, oregano, pepper and salt (if desired).
3. Bring to the boil and add mussels.
4. Cover and cook until shells open (this takes only a few minutes).
5. Serve in bowls with crusty bread.

Nutrition data per serve: 723 kJ (173 cal), CHO 6 g, Protein 25 g, Fat 5 g.

Preparation time: 15-20 minutes. Cooking equipment: large saucepan.

Salmon Mornay

Serves: 4

440 g (15 oz) can salmon
4 spring onions (shallots), chopped
4 tbsp lemon juice
2 stalks celery, finely chopped
2 tbsp freshly grated parmesan cheese
1 quantity Cheese Sauce (see recipe, page 155)
garnish: 2 hard-boiled eggs, chopped

Method:

1. Mix salmon, chopped spring onions (shallots), lemon juice and celery in casserole.
2. Add parmesan cheese to sauce and pour over salmon mixture. Mix well.
3. Bake for 30 minutes. Alternatively, cover and microwave on 'medium' for 12-14 minutes, and then let stand, covered, for 5 minutes before serving.
4. Sprinkle with chopped eggs and serve.

Nutrition data per serve: 1219 kJ (291 cal), CHO 12 g, Protein 32 g, Fat 13 g.

Preparation time: 45 minutes. Cooking equipment: mornay dish or shallow casserole. Oven temperature: 180°C (350°F).

Seafood Cannelloni

Serves: 4

2 tsp olive oil
2 cloves garlic, crushed
2 medium onions, finely chopped
½ cup tomato paste
2 cups water
2 tsp lemon juice
½ tsp ground thyme
1 tsp ground basil
salt to taste (optional)
200 g (7 oz) white fish, cut into small chunks
150 g (5 oz) shelled prawns, coarsely chopped
100 g (3 oz) scallops, coarsely chopped
½ cup fresh wholemeal breadcrumbs
2 tbsp chopped parsley
2 tbsp dry white wine
ground black pepper to taste
1 egg, lightly beaten
12 lightly cooked cannelloni shells (to make handling easier)
½ cup grated low-fat block cheese

This is a recipe for special occasions. For a family meal, you may like to omit scallops and prawns and replace them with 500 g (1 lb) of minced white fish.

Method:

1. Heat oil in frying pan and sauté 1 clove garlic and 1 onion until tender.
2. Add tomato paste, water, lemon juice, ¼ tsp thyme, ½ tsp basil and salt. Set aside.
3. Combine remaining garlic, onion, thyme and basil with fish, prawns, scallops, breadcrumbs, parsley, wine, pepper and egg.
4. Spoon fish mixture into cannelloni shells, and arrange in a shallow casserole.
5. Pour tomato mixture over cannelloni shells and sprinkle with cheese.
6. Bake for 30 minutes until sauce is hot and bubbling.

Nutrition data per serve: 1747 kJ (417 cal), CHO 40 g, Protein 38 g, Fat 11 g.

Preparation time: 1 hour. Cooking equipment: frying pan, shallow casserole. Oven temperature: 180°C (350°F).

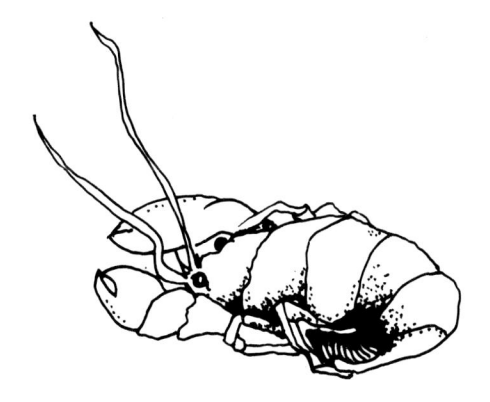

Meats and Poultry

Pork Tango

Serves: 4

1 cup boiling water
½ cup dried apricots
1 tbsp dried currants
500 g (1 lb) pork scotch fillet, trimmed of fat
1 beaten egg
2 tsp sesame seeds
2 tbsp fresh breadcrumbs
1 clove garlic, finely chopped or minced (optional)
2 tbsp mango chutney or Fresh Mango Pickle (recipe page 163)
1 tbsp brandy
¼ cup canned evaporated skim milk

This is a favourite recipe. The brandy loses its alcohol during heating, but rounds out the lovely fruity sauce. Leave it out if you prefer. You can substitute half a cup of crushed pineapple for the apricots, but remember to reduce the water to half a cup.

Method:

1. Pour boiling water over apricots and currants in a bowl, and stand for half an hour.
2. Roll pork first in egg and then in a mixture of sesame seeds, breadcrumbs and garlic until well coated.
3. Place in roasting pan and bake, uncovered, in a preheated oven for 45 minutes.
4. While meat is cooking, heat apricots in a saucepan with the currants and the water in which they were soaked.
5. Simmer gently until water is almost absorbed.
6. Add chutney and brandy and stir until the sauce returns to the simmer.
7. Pour evaporated skim milk in a heat-resistant bowl and gradually stir in the hot apricot mixture (this method will prevent the milk curdling).
8. Return to saucepan and reheat without boiling.
9. To test if meat is cooked, pierce with a skewer. Juice should be clear.
10. Cut meat into eight slices, arrange two slices on each serving plate and spoon sauce over, distributing apricot halves evenly.

To store: both meat and sauce will keep for two days if well covered in the refrigerator. They can be served cold, in which case store meat in one piece and slice thinly just before serving, using the cold sauce as an accompaniment.

Nutrition data per serve: 1057 kJ (252 cal), CHO 22 g, Protein 34 g, Fat 4 g.
Preparation time: 1 hour. Cooking equipment: roasting pan, small saucepan, heat-proof bowl. Oven temperature: 200°C (400°F).

Foreground: Chick Pea Savoury. On the round platter, left, assorted pumpernickel savouries, right, Vegetable Samosas, Wholemeal Salmon Slices in the centre, and Dolmades at the back.

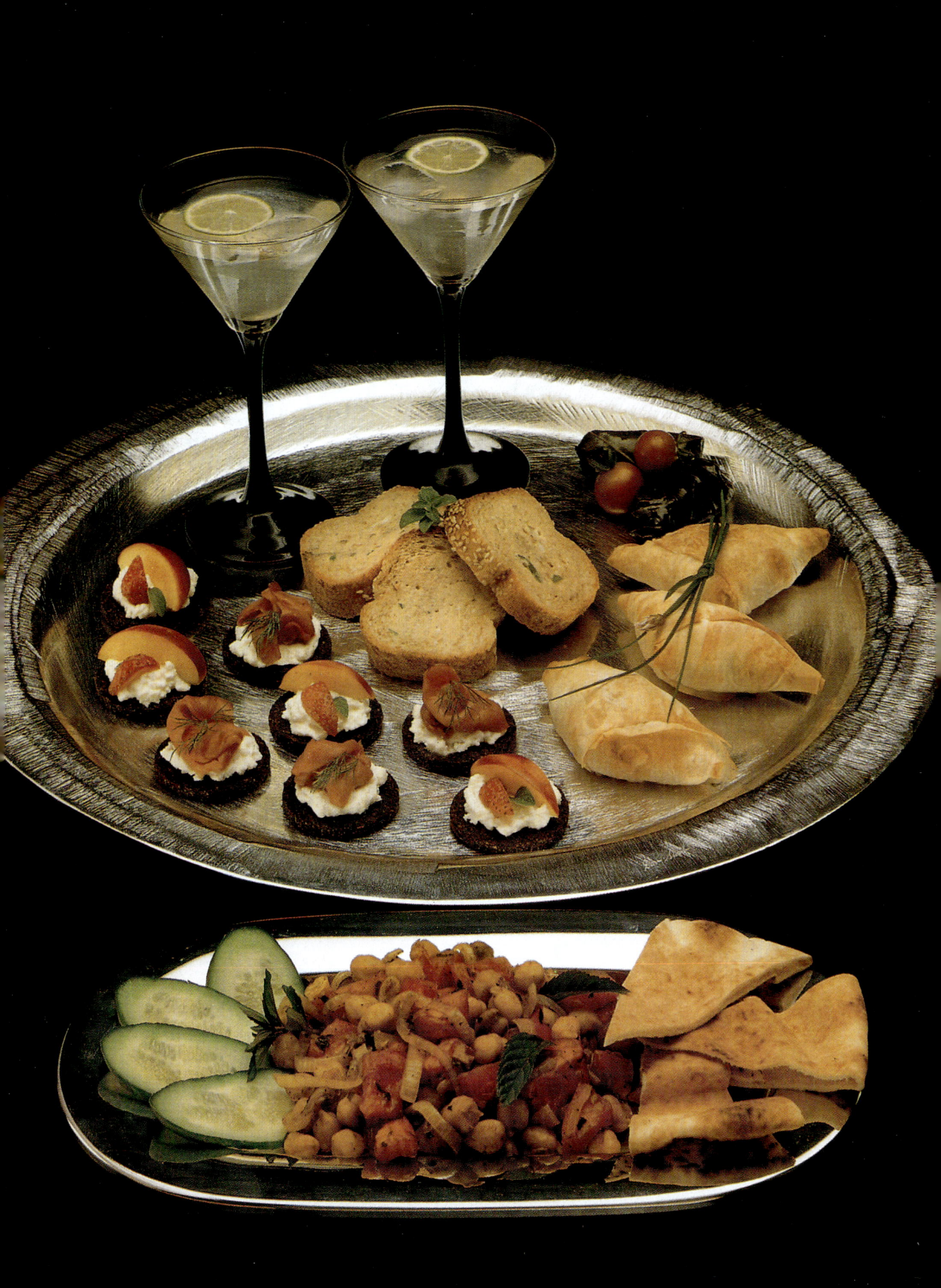

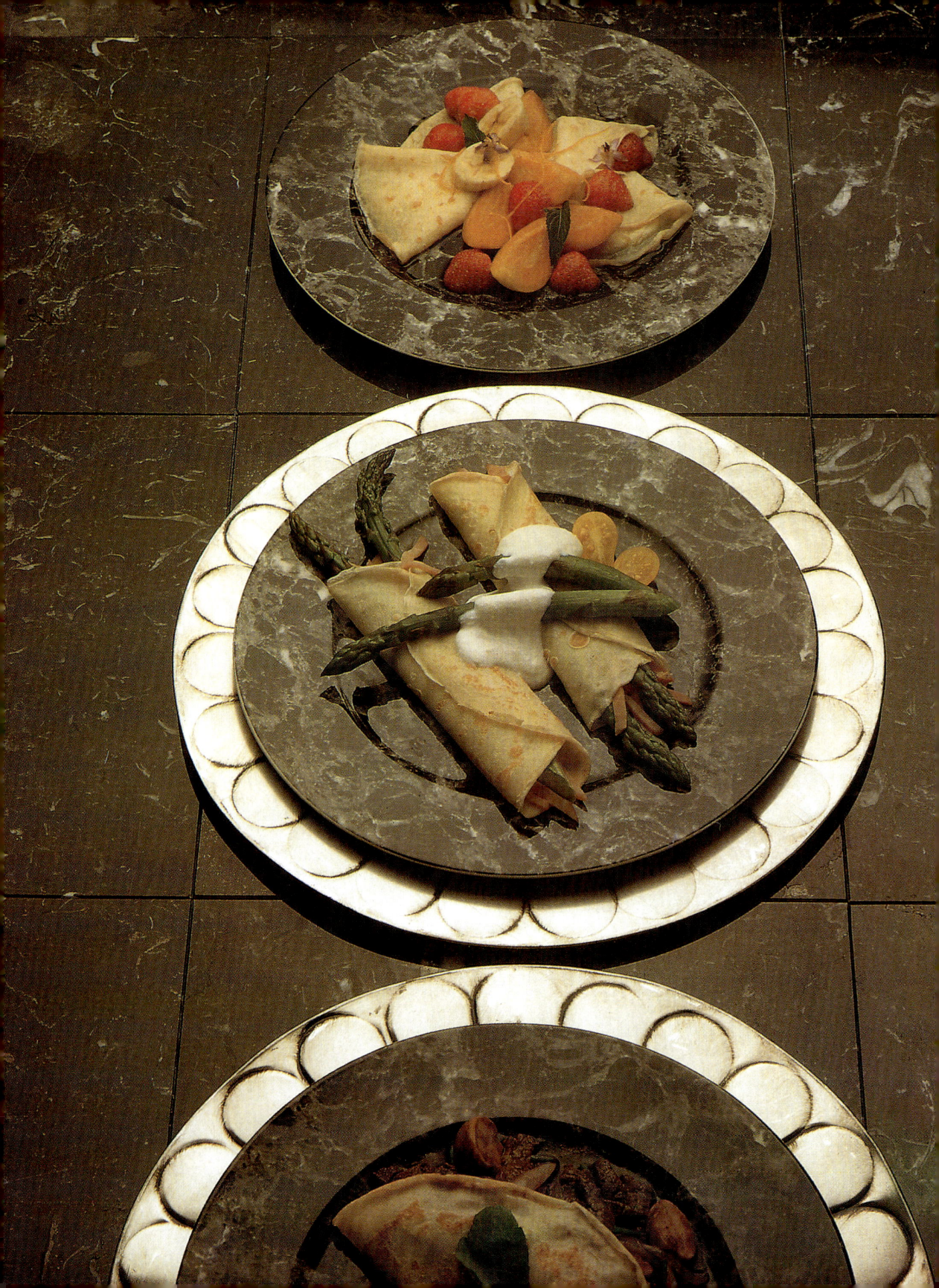

Chinese Stir-fry Pork

Serves: 4-5

500 g (1 lb) pork fillet
1 tbsp polyunsaturated oil
½ tsp ginger grated
1 clove garlic, crushed
   pinch Chinese five spice powder
1 cup small broccoli florets
1 cup small cauliflower florets
½ green capsicum (bell pepper), diced
2 medium carrots, cut into matchsticks (julienne)
3 spring onions (shallots), chopped
16-20 snow peas
10-12 button mushrooms, sliced
2 stalks celery sliced diagonally
1 apple, cut into slices
¼ cucumber, cut into slices
1 tbsp soy sauce
1 tbsp honey
1 tbsp tomato sauce
1½ tbsp cornflour (cornstarch)
1 cup Chicken Stock (recipe, page 72)

The secret of a successful stir-fry is to have all the ingredients prepared before you begin cooking, and then to cook them swiftly so that they reach the table still crisp and alive with colour.

Method:

1. Prepare pork fillet by slicing thinly at an angle.
2. Heat oil in pan until very hot. Add pork, ginger, garlic and five spice. Stir-fry for 3-5 minutes.
3. Add broccoli, cauliflower, capsicum (bell pepper) and carrots. Stir-fry 1-2 minutes, making sure that nothing is allowed to over-cook and become limp.
4. Now add the rest of the vegetables and continue stir-frying over high heat for another 1-2 minutes.
5. In a bowl, combine soy sauce, honey, tomato sauce, cornflour (cornstarch) and chicken stock. Add mixture to the chicken and vegetables, bring to the boil, cover, turn down the heat and simmer 2-3 minutes only.
6. Serve on a bed of boiled brown rice.

To vary: replace the pork with chicken or veal.

Nutrition data per serve (based on 4 serves): 1329 kJ (318 cal), CHO 25 g, Protein 31 g, Fat 11 g.

Preparation time: 45 minutes. Cooking equipment: large saucepan or wok.

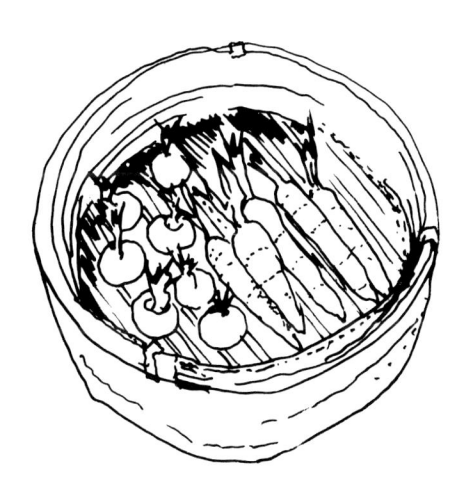

Crêpes with fillings: foreground, Steak and Onion, centre, Ham and Asparagus, delicious Flambéed Fruit at the top.

Eat & Enjoy   Meats and Poultry

Malaysian Fried Rice Noodles (Char Kway Teow)

Serves: 4

1 tbsp peanut oil
1 clove garlic, finely chopped
2 small onions, sliced
1–2 fresh chillies, deseeded and chopped
100 g (3 oz) barbecue pork, lean, cut into strips
150 g (5 oz) small green prawns, shelled and deveined
150 g (5 oz) calamari (squid) rings
1 cup bean sprouts
300 g (10 oz) fresh rice noodles (kway teow)
2 tbsp soy sauce
2 tsp oyster sauce
pepper to taste
2 eggs, beaten
garnish: 3 spring onions (shallots), chopped

Method:

1. Heat ½ oil in wok and fry garlic, onion and chilli until soft.
2. Add pork, prawns and calamari and continue cooking for 2–3 minutes or until seafood is cooked.
3. Add bean sprouts and toss.
4. Remove mixture from wok.
5. Add remaining oil to wok, heat and then add noodles. Toss gently until heated.
6. Add soy and oyster sauces and pepper and toss to mix.
7. Add eggs and stir till set.
8. Return seafood mixture to wok, mix in well.
9. Serve hot garnished with chopped spring onions (shallots).

Note: Chinese grocery stores sell fresh rice noodles as 'sa hor fun'.

Nutrition data per serve : 1894 kJ (453 cal), CHO 48 g, Protein 34 g, Fat 14 g.

Preparation time: 20 minutes. Cooking Equipment: 1 wok or large saucepan.

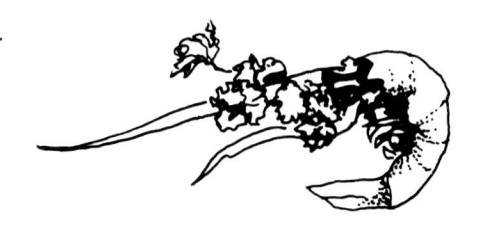

Meatloaf with Spicy Barbecue Sauce

Serves: 4

500 g (1 lb) minced lean beef
3 slices of wholemeal bread, crumbed
1 onion, finely chopped
2 tsp Curry Powder (recipe, page 164)
1 tbsp chopped parsley
1 egg
½ cup skim or low-fat milk
Sauce:
½ cup water
½ cup tomato sauce
¼ cup Worcestershire sauce
2 tbsp vinegar
1 tsp instant coffee
juice of 1 lemon
1 tbsp cornflour (cornstarch)
1 tbsp water

This meatloaf cooks in its own luscious dark, piquant sauce.

Method:

1. Combine minced steak, breadcrumbs, onion, curry powder, parsley and egg.
2. Stir until mixture is well combined.
3. Add milk and continue stirring until mixture is smooth.
4. Shape meat mixture into a loaf and place in baking dish.
5. Bake in preheated oven for 30 minutes, or microwave, covered, on 'medium' for 20 minutes.
6. Remove from oven or microwave and drain off any fat.
7. In a saucepan, combine all sauce ingredients, except the cornflour (cornstarch) and 1 tbsp of water, bring slowly to boil, reduce heat and simmer for 5 minutes.
8. Pour sauce over meat and return to oven or microwave.
9. Bake for a further 20-30 minutes, basting frequently with sauce, or microwave on 'medium' for a further 20 minutes.
10. Mix cornflour (cornstarch) and water to a smooth paste. Remove meatloaf to a serving plate and slice.
11. Add cornflour (cornstarch) mixture to the sauce in the baking dish and bring back to the boil, stirring constantly until thickened.
12. Pour thickened sauce over the meatloaf. Serve hot with vegetables or cold with salad.

To store: keep in airtight container or cover with plastic film in refrigerator for up to two days. You can also freeze it in an airtight container.

Nutrition data per serve: 1210 kJ (289 cal), CHO 24 g, Protein 34 g, Fat 7 g.
Preparation time: 1 hour. Cooking equipment: baking dish, medium saucepan.
Oven temperature: 180°C (350°F).

Meatballs in Tomato Sauce

Serves: 4

500 g (1 lb) lean minced beef
1 tbsp chopped parsley
1 tsp curry powder
3 slices wholemeal bread, crumbed
1 beaten egg
2½ tsp water
2 medium onions, finely chopped
425 g (15 oz) can tomatoes
1 tbsp tomato paste
½ tsp dried oregano
ground black pepper to taste
garnish: parsley

All you need to is to make the meatballs, prepare potatoes, brown rice, crushed wheat or noodles, make a mixed salad, and you have a perfect meal.

Method:

1. Combine beef, parsley, curry and breadcrumbs in a bowl.
2. Add the egg and water to bind the mixture.
3. Roll into 16 equal balls.
4. Place in a baking dish and cook in oven at 180°C (350°F) for 30 minutes.
5. Heat saucepan with 2 teaspoons of water and lightly cook the onion until translucent, stirring frequently.
6. Add tomatoes, tomato paste and oregano.
7. Reduce heat and simmer 10 minutes.
8. Add pepper to taste.
9. Pour sauce over meatballs, replace in oven and reduce heat to 160°C (325°F).
10. Bake for an additional 30 minutes.
11. Serve, garnished with parsley.

To store: cover and refrigerate for up to three days.

Microwave method

Follow Steps 1 to 3 as above. Then preheat a browning dish on 'high' for 6-7 minutes. Place the meatballs on the browning dish and cook them on 'high' for 4-6 minutes, turning the meatballs three times during the cooking process. Remove the meatballs to a shallow microwave dish and set aside. Place the onions in a bowl and cook them on 'high' until they are translucent. Add the tomatoes, tomato paste and oregano to the onions. Cook the onion mixture on 'high' for 5 minutes. Add pepper to taste. Pour the sauce over the meatballs, and cook on 'medium' for a further 15 minutes.

Nutrition data per serve: 1016 kJ (243 cal), CHO 13 g, Protein 33 g, Fat 7 g.
Preparation time: 1 ½ hours. Cooking equipment: baking dish, saucepan.
Oven temperature: 180°C (350°F) then 160°C (325°F)

Beef Curry

Serves: 4

500 g (1 lb) lean beef (topside, round, bolar blade)
ground black pepper
2 tsp oil (optional)
1 large onion peeled and chopped
2 potatoes scrubbed and chopped
½ cup skinned and chopped pumpkin
½ cup peeled and chopped sweet potato (yam)
2 zucchini cut into chunks
1 tsp dried coriander
1 tsp dried cumin
½ tsp dried cardamom
2 tsp mustard seeds
½–1 tsp dried ground chillies
2 tsp finely chopped or minced fresh ginger
2 tsp finely chopped or minced garlic
1 cup water
pinch of salt to taste (optional)

This dish is best when prepared the day before eating, to allow the flavour to develop. A pinch of salt helps bring out the taste of the spices, but use discretion.

Method:

1. Trim any fat from meat. Cut into 2-3 cm (1 in) cubes and sprinkle with pepper.
2. In a frying pan, dry fry (or sauté in 2 tsp of hot oil) until browned on all sides. Set aside in a bowl.
3. In the same frying pan, sauté the vegetables and set aside with the meat.
4. Now add to the frying pan the dry spices and cook for 3-4 minutes over medium heat to release the fragrance, then add the ginger and garlic.
5. Add water and stir the pan juices well.
6. Return meat and vegetables to pan, add salt if desired, and stir to combine the flavours.
7. Spoon into casserole, cover and cook in oven for approximately 1½–2 hours until meat is tender.
8. Serve with brown rice and the accompaniments suggested below.

To store: cover and refrigerate for up to four days.

Nutrition data per serve: 1169 kJ (279 cal), CHO 18 g, Protein 31 g, Fat 9 g.

Preparation time: 2 ½ hours. Cooking equipment: large frying pan, casserole. Oven temperature: 200°C (400°F).

Curry Accompaniments

Fresh Mango Pickle (recipe, page 163), pineapple with paw paw, sultanas with coconut, and diced apple are excellent with curry.

Tomato Mint Salad

Mix 1 ripe tomato, finely chopped, with 2 spring onions (shallots) sliced and 2 tsp chopped fresh mint. Chill until ready to serve.

Nutrition data per serve: 36 kJ (9 cal), CHO 2 g, Protein 1 g, Fat 0 g.

Banana-yoghurt Relish

Slice 2 firm bananas and sprinkle them with 1 tbsp of shredded coconut. Spoon ¼ cup of low-fat yoghurt over bananas and combine. Chill until ready to serve.

Nutrition data per serve: 389 kJ (93 cal), CHO 17 g, Protein 2 g, Fat 2 g.

Cucumber and Yoghurt

Combine piece of cucumber (about 10cm/4 in long) with 2 tsp lemon juice and ½ tsp. of mustard seeds. Spoon ¼ cup of low-fat natural yoghurt over the cucumber and combine with yoghurt. Chill until ready to serve.

Nutrition data per serve: 46 kJ (11 cal), CHO 1 g, Protein 1 g, Fat 0 g.

Skewered Lamb

*Serves: 4
(3 skewers each)*

1 cup low-fat natural yoghurt
3 tbsp French mustard
¼ tsp ground thyme
¼ tsp ground oregano
2 sprigs rosemary
2 bay leaves
500 g (1 lb) diced lean lamb

Baked jacket potatoes and a large mixed salad makes this a memorable meal.

Method:

1. Mix yoghurt with mustard and herbs, add lamb and stir well.
2. Stand for 10-12 hours.
3. Remove rosemary and bay leaves
4. Thread meat onto skewers, grill or barbecue until cooked.

Nutrition data per serve: 744 kJ (178 cal), CHO 3 g, Protein 30 g, Fat 5 g.

Preparation time: 1 hour, plus 10-12 hours marinading time. Cooking equipment: 12 wooden skewers (soaked in water for 1 hour before using to prevent burning), grill or barbecue.

Meat à la Pizzaiola

Serves: 4

500 g (1 lb) lean beef fillet
1 tsp oil
1 clove garlic, crushed
½ cup sliced mushrooms
2 large tomatoes, peeled and chopped
2 spring onions (shallots), chopped
4 leaves fresh basil, roughly chopped, or ¼ tsp dried basil
freshly ground black pepper
salt to taste (optional)
garnish: spring onion (shallot)

Although beef fillet is a relatively expensive cut of meat, in this recipe you use only half a kilogram to feed four people. The meat cooks quickly, so there is little shrinkage and as fillet is lean, there is no waste. The recipe will work just as successfully if you use veal, pork or chicken. Add a few drops of tabasco sauce if you want to make the sauce more piquant.

Method:

1. Cut the meat into thin strips, about 1 cm x 5 cm (½ in x 2 in).
2. Brush oil over the base of a heavy frying pan and heat the pan over medium-high heat.
3. When hot, toss in the meat and stir-fry until well sealed and browned (approximately 2–3 minutes).
4. Set the meat aside on a warm plate and continue as follows. To the hot frying pan add the garlic and the mushrooms and stir-fry for a further few seconds until the mushrooms are lightly cooked.
5. Add the chopped tomatoes, spring onions (shallots), fresh basil, pepper and salt, and bring to a simmer. Now return the meat to the sauce and simmer for about 5 minutes, or until the meat is cooked and the dish is hot.
6. Finally, spoon the meat and sauce onto a bed of rice or noodles, garnish with spring onion (shallot) and serve.

To store: cover and refrigerate for up to three days.

Nutrition data per serve: 713 kJ (170 cal), CHO 3 g, Protein 28 g, Fat 5 g.
Preparation time: 15 minutes. Cooking equipment: large saucepan, large frying pan.

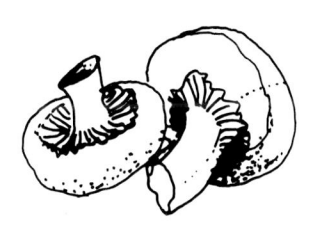

Pickled Beef

Serves: 8

1 kg (2 lb) piece of beef topside
12 whole cloves
1 cup wine vinegar (red or white)
1 cup red wine
2 tsp brown sugar
½ tsp prepared mustard
½ tsp mustard seeds
½ tsp finely chopped garlic
½ tsp peppercorns
1 medium onion, chopped

You may never have considered making your own pickled beef, so this delicious recipe may be an eye-opener. The commercial product tends to be full of salt and saltpetre which is not desirable.

Method:

1. Trim any fat from meat.
2. Stick cloves into meat, evenly distributed.
3. Place meat in a bowl large enough to hold it snugly.
4. Combine vinegar, wine, sugar, mustard, mustard seeds, garlic, peppercorns and onions and pour over meat.
5. Cover tightly and refrigerate for three days, turning once or twice each day.
6. Remove meat from bowl and place in large saucepan.
7. Strain marinating liquid through a sieve into smaller saucepan. Bring to boil and strain over meat.
8. Cover, bring to boil, immediately lower the heat and simmer gently until meat is cooked through (about 1 hour).
9. Serve hot with boiled or mashed potatoes and cooked red cabbage, or cold with bread or with a salad.

To store: cover and refrigerate for up to one week. Excellent to take camping.

Nutrition data per serve: 658 kJ (157 cal), CHO 2 g, Protein 27 g, Fat 5 g.

Preparation time: 1½ hours plus 3 days marinating. Cooking equipment: saucepan, large saucepan with lid.

Chilli Con Carne

Serves: 4

500 g (1 lb) topside, cubed
2 tsp oil (optional)
1 large onion, chopped
4 large tomatoes, chopped

This dish is equally successful if you use lean beef mince instead of topside.

Method:

1. Trim off all fat from topside and cut into 2-3 cm (1 in) cubes.
2. Brush frying pan with oil and brown meat or dry fry meat until well browned.

150 g (5 oz) can tomato paste

1 cup water and ¼ cup water

425 g (15 oz) can red kidney beans

2 tsp tabasco sauce

¼ tsp ground black pepper

1 tbsp cornflour (cornstarch)

3. Spoon into casserole.
4. Add onion to frying pan and sauté until lightly browned.
5. Add tomatoes and cook over medium heat until soft. Stir occasionally.
6. Stir in tomato paste and 1 cup water. Mix well.
7. Rinse kidney beans, drain well, and add to the mixture.
8. Add tabasco sauce and pepper, pour over meat and combine.
9. Mix cornflour (cornstarch) with ¼ cup water. When smooth stir into mixture.
10. Cover casserole, cook in oven until meat is tender (approximately 1½ hours).

To store: cover and refrigerate for up to three days.

Nutrition data per serve: 1485 kJ (355 cal), CHO 34 g, Protein 39 g, Fat 7 g.

Preparation time: 2 hours. Cooking equipment: large frying pan or electric frying pan, lidded casserole. Oven temperature: 180°C (350°F).

Steak and Black Bean Sauce

Serves: 4

2 tsp oil

500 g (1 lb) fillet or lean rump steak, trimmed of fat

1 medium onion, peeled and quartered

¼ cup coarsely chopped green capsicum (bell pepper)

¼ cup coarsely chopped red capsicum (bell pepper)

1 medium carrot, cut into rings

1 quantity Black Bean Sauce (recipe page 157)

None of the ingredients in this recipe should be cooked for more than a few minutes. At the table, the vegetables should still be crisp and have their true vibrant colour.

Method:

1. Brush oil over the base of a frying pan or wok and heat over high heat.
2. Slice steak into very thin strips 3-4 cm (2-3 in) long and ½ cm (⅓ in) wide. Sauté quickly for about 3 minutes.
3. Add vegetables and stir-fry for a further 2 minutes.
4. Add black bean sauce, cover and simmer gently for 5 minutes.
5. Serve with boiled brown rice.

Nutrition data per serve: 1031 kJ (246 cal), CHO 6, Protein 32 g, Fat 11 g.

Preparation time: ½ hour. Cooking equipment: frying pan or wok.

Leg of Lamb with Garlic and Mustard

Serves: 8

1.5 kg (3½ lb) leg of lamb
2 cloves garlic, crushed
1 tsp dried rosemary
2 tbsp soy sauce
3 tbsp prepared French mustard
2 tbsp cornflour (cornstarch)
1 cup water
garnish: sprig of rosemary or mint

Method:

1. Trim all fat from the lamb, place the lamb in baking dish.
2. Combine garlic, rosemary, soy sauce and mustard and spread over leg of lamb.
3. Bake, covered, in a preheated oven until cooked to your taste.
4. Remove leg of lamb from dish and carve.
5. Pour or skim the fat from meat juices.
6. Blend cornflour (cornstarch) with a little water to form a smooth paste, and add to the meat juices.
7. Heat until thickened, stirring constantly to keep the gravy smooth, and pour over slices of lamb.

To store: covered and refrigerate for up to three days.

Nutrition data per serve: 671 kJ (160 cal), CHO 2 g, Protein 27 g, Fat 5 g.
Preparation time: 1 ¾–2 hours. Cooking equipment: baking dish.
Oven temperature: 180°C (350°F).

Baked Fillet with Cherry Sauce

Serves: 8

1 kg (2 lb) eye fillet of beef, trimmed of visible fat
2 tsp chopped, fresh oregano or 1 tsp dried
3 small sprigs fresh rosemary or 1 tsp dried
1 quantity Cherry Sauce (recipe, page 154)
garnish: 4 sprigs oregano or rosemary

Eye fillet is an expensive cut, but for a special occasion it is worth it. Remember, too, that there is no waste and, in this recipe, you can serve eight with only a kilogram (two pounds) of fillet.

Method:

1. Place the beef on a large piece of aluminium foil.
2. Sprinkle with oregano and rosemary and wrap beef.
3. Place in a baking dish, bake for 30 minutes in a preheated oven.
4. Uncover and bake for a further 15 minutes.
5. Remove from oven, pour juices into cherry sauce. Loosely cover meat with foil and let stand in a warm place.
6. Heat sauce.
7. Cut beef into thick slices and serve topped with cherry sauce and garnished with a sprig of oregano or rosemary.

Nutrition data per serve: 728 kJ (174 cal), CHO 6 g, Protein 27 g, Fat 5 g.
Preparation time: approximately 1 hour. Cooking equipment: baking dish.
Oven temperature: 210°C (425°F).

Indian Lamb in Spinach Sauce

Serves: 4

6 ripe tomatoes or 440 g (14 oz) canned tomatoes
1 tbsp polyunsaturated vegetable oil
2 cloves garlic, finely chopped
2 tsp fresh ginger, finely chopped
2 fresh green or red chillies, finely chopped or 1 tsp minced chilli paste
salt to taste
500 g (1 lb) lean lamb, diced
1/4 tsp each of ground cumin, coriander, cinnamon, cloves and turmeric
3 bunches fresh spinach, finely chopped, or 750 g (1.5 lb) frozen spinach, thawed

Method:

1. Blend tomatoes in a food processor.
2. Heat oil in saucepan, add garlic, ginger, chillies and salt. Cook, stirring, for 2 minutes.
3. Add lamb, mix well, cover and cook over low heat for 30–40 minutes or until lamb is tender.
4. Add tomatoes and cook for a further 10 minutes.
5. Add spices and simmer gently for 10 minutes.
6. Add spinach and simmer for a further 4 minutes.

Ideal served with Dry Curry of Potato, Eggplant and Pea (recipe, page 136).

Nutrition data per serve: 889 kJ (212 cal), CHO 3 g, Protein 29 g, Fat 9 g.

Preparation time: 1½-hours. Cooking equipment: 1 large, heavy based saucepan with lid.

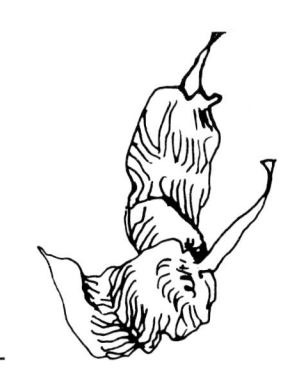

Mogul Lamb

Serves: 6

6 large ripe tomatoes or 440 g (14 oz) canned tomatoes, chopped
½ cup water
4 cloves garlic, finely chopped
2 tsp ginger, finely chopped
3 fresh chillies, finely chopped
1 tsp ground black pepper
½ tsp each of ground cardamom, cloves, fennel, cinnamon, fenugreek
4 tbsp fresh coriander leaves, chopped
1 tbsp each of fresh basil, dill and mint, chopped
salt to taste
1 x 1.5 kg (3 lb) leg lamb, boned and trimmed of all visible fat

Method:

1. Place tomatoes, garlic, ginger, chillies and pepper into a saucepan and simmer, stirring occasionally for 15 minutes.
2. Add all other ingredients but the lamb, mix well and set aside.
3. Place lamb into a casserole dish, spread well with tomato mixture, cover and stand for 20 minutes in refrigerator to marinate.
4. Place uncovered in oven and bake for 1¼ hours or until cooked.

Suitable to accompany Spiced Rice with Peas (recipe, page 140).

Variation: use 1 kg (2 lb) lean diced lamb or fillets and reduce cooking time accordingly.

Nutrition data per serve: 891 kJ (213 cal), CHO 2 g, Protein 37 g, Fat 6 g.

Preparation time: 1¾ hours. Cooking equipment: 1 medium saucepan, 1 large casserole or oven-proof dish. Oven temperature: 180°C (350°F).

Opposite:
Foreground left: fresh lychees, Beef and Black Bean Sauce at the right, Gado Gado served with Chicken and Saté Sauce at centre, and a steamer of brown rice with Hot and Sour Soup below it.

Overleaf:
Front right: Chicken Enchiladas, a Tossed Salad at centre with Mexicale Pie with Corn Dumplings beside it, and a cool Golden Fruit Flummery at the top.

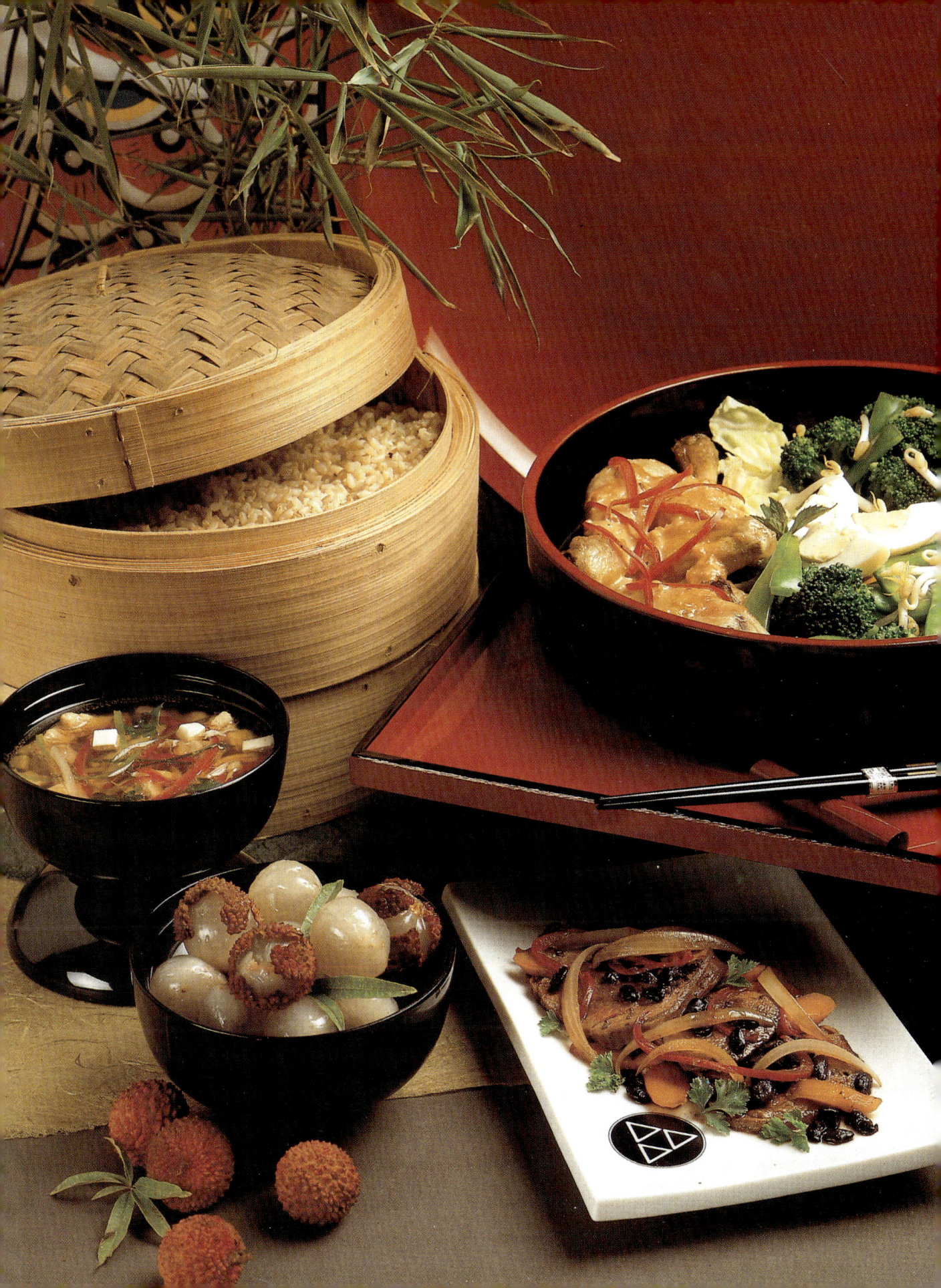

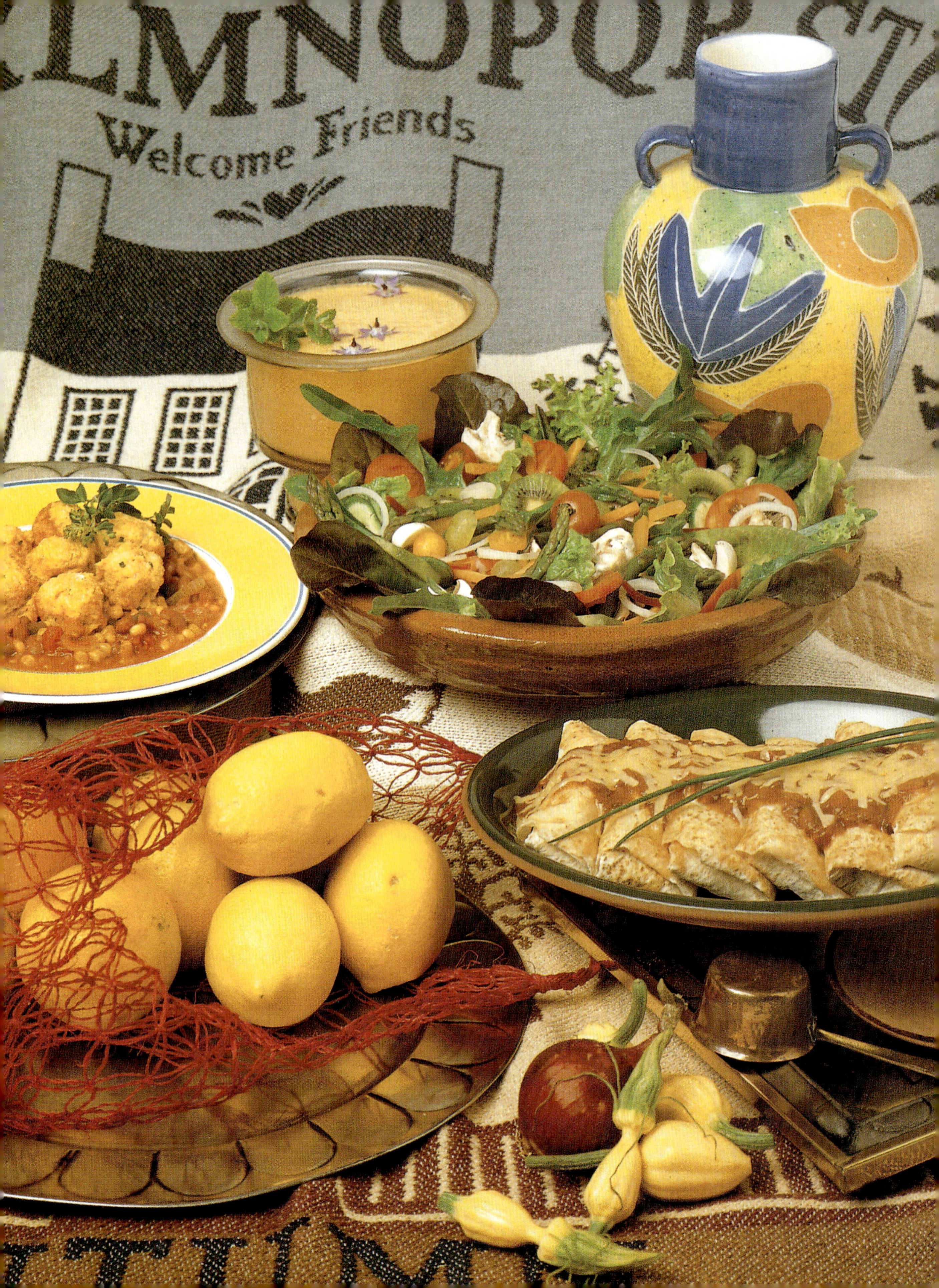
LMNOPQR STU
Welcome Friends

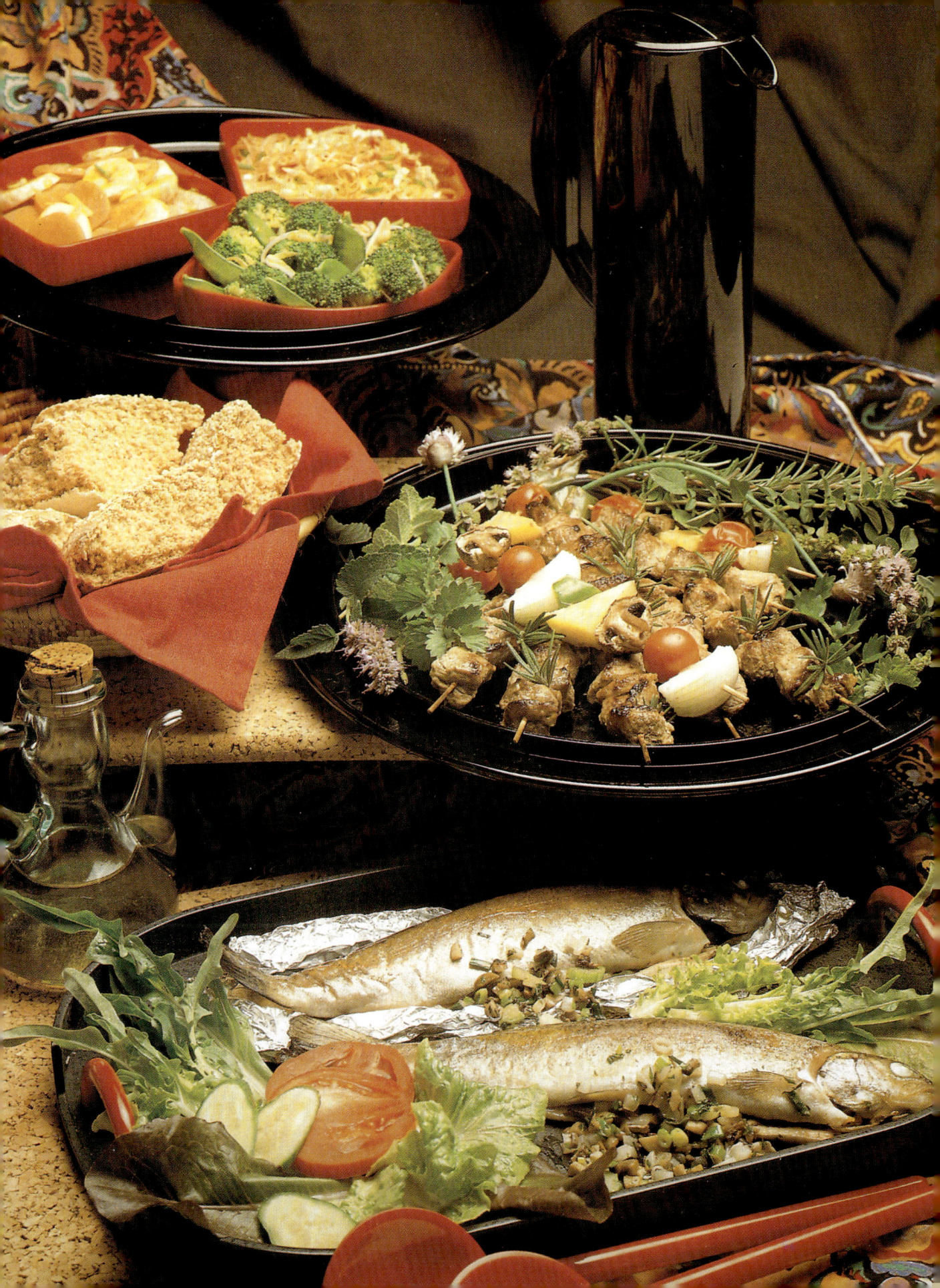

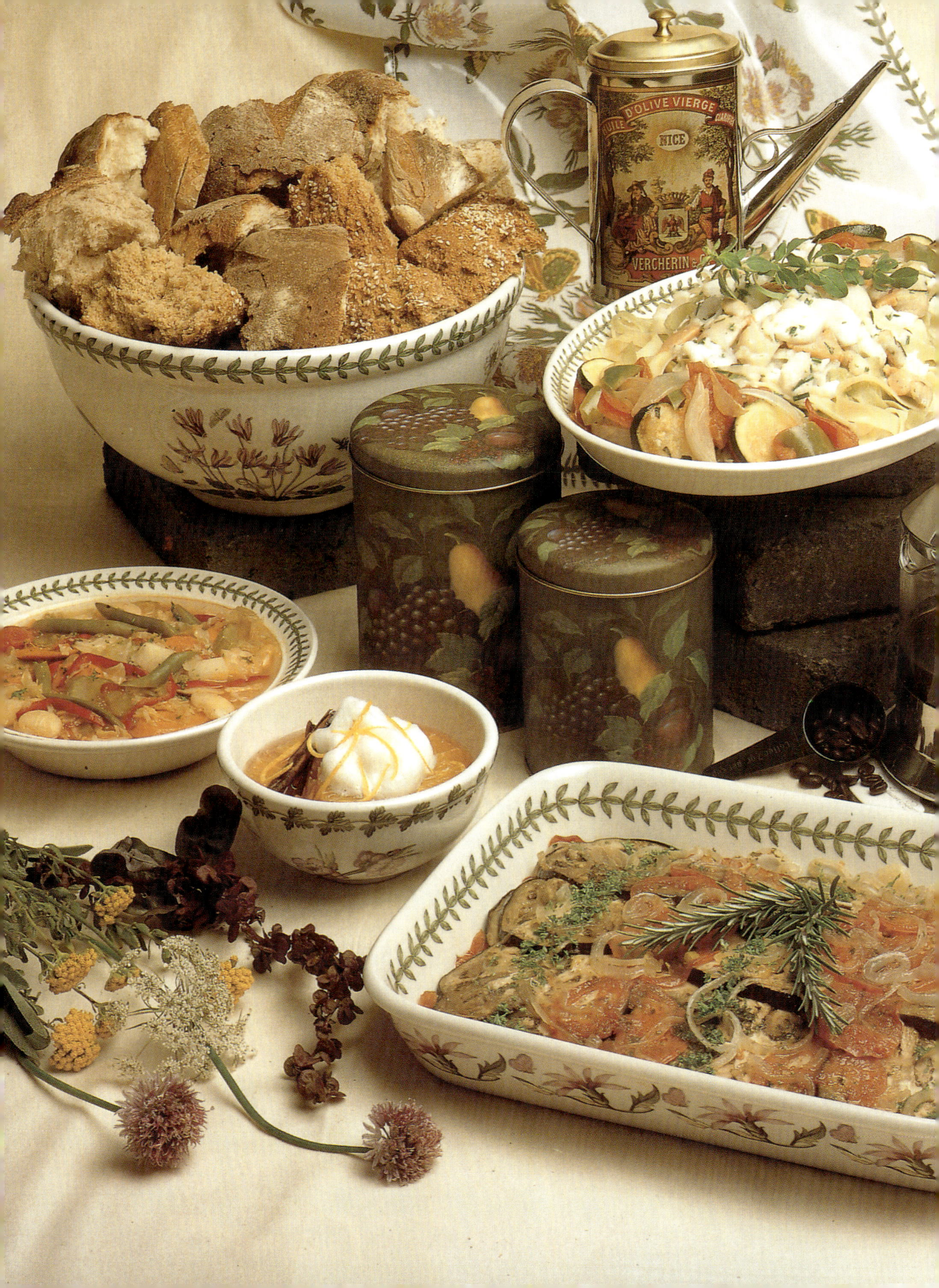
HUILE
D'OLIVE VIERGE
NICE
VERCHERIN

Veal Mango

Serves: 4

Sauce:
2 small or 1 large mango
1 cup dry white wine
3 tbsp mango chutney or Fresh Mango Pickle (recipe page 163)
4 tbsp chopped spring onions (shallots)
Veal:
1 tsp oil
4 lean veal schnitzels
2 tbsp water
garnish: 4 spring onions (shallots)

This is a wonderful recipe that is very easy to prepare and yet looks and tastes good enough for a special occasion. Simple boiled rice and a crisp green salad round out the meal. Pork schnitzel or chicken fillets make an excellent and economical substitute for the veal.

Method:

1. Make the sauce. Peel the mangoes. Cut away and roughly slice the flesh.
2. Place the mango flesh in a saucepan. Add the white wine and pickle or chutney. Bring to the boil, reduce heat and simmer until the sauce has reduced by half, about 15 minutes.
3. If you want a smooth sauce, purée the hot fruit mixture in a food processor or blender, or force through a sieve. Return to saucepan.
4. Add the chopped spring onions (shallots). Return to the boil, reduce heat and simmer for a further 2-3 minutes.
5. Prepare the veal schnitzels. While the sauce is simmering, at Step 2, brush a large frying pan with the oil and heat over medium-high heat.
6. Fry the schnitzels, turning occasionally, for approximately 10 minutes until browned on both sides.
7. Remove the cooked schnitzels from the pan. Add the 2 tbsp of water to the pan, as well as the sauce. Heat, stirring constantly, for about 3 minutes.
8. Arrange the schnitzels on individual dinner plates. Spoon over the sauce and garnish with the whole spring onions (shallots).

Nutrition data per serve: 734 kJ (175 cal), CHO 9 g, Protein 28 g, Fat 3 g.
Preparation time: 40 minutes. Cooking equipment: saucepan, frying pan.

Previous page:
Foreground: Vegetable Stuffed Trout, centre right a platter of Skewered Lamb and Vegetables en Brochette beside a basket of Wholemeal Damper. At the top Coleslaw, Curried Sweet Potato and Banana Salad and Broccoli, Beanshoots and Snowpeas with Lemon.

Opposite:
Foreground: Eggplant Neapolitan, centre, Spiced Oranges with Creamy Whipped Topping, to the left, Minestrone below a bowl of crusty bread. Back right Pasta Marinara served with Zucchini Creole.

Caesar's Chicken

Serves: 4

1 No. 12 or 800 g (1¾ lb) chicken
1½ cups water
2-3 sprigs fresh dill or ¼ tsp dried dill
¼ cup vinegar
1 small leek, thickly sliced
Sauce:
200 g (7 oz) pitted dates
1 chicken stock cube
1 tsp caraway seeds
½ tsp dried coriander
¼ tsp dried cardamom
2 tsp fresh mint, chopped
½ tsp finely chopped or minced fresh ginger
2 tsp Plum Sauce (recipe, page 163) or commercial plum sauce
3 tbsp vinegar
1 cup water

The touch of sweetness and the thickness of the sauce in this Middle Eastern dish come from the addition of dates.

Method:

1. Cut chicken into pieces, discarding wings, skin and fat.
2. Place chicken in saucepan with water, dill, vinegar and leek.
3. Cover, bring to the boil, immediately turn down the heat and simmer gently for 30 minutes.
4. Chop dates and place in second saucepan. Add stock cube, caraway, coriander, cardamom, mint, ginger, plum sauce, vinegar and water.
5. Cook, stirring gently until the dates have broken down and the sauce thickens.
6. Lift chicken out of cooking broth, place in casserole or baking dish, pour sauce over, cover with foil and bake for 15-20 minutes.

To store: cover and refrigerate for up to two days.

Nutrition data per serve: 1306 kJ (312 cal), CHO 33 g, Protein 32 g, Fat 6 g.

Preparation time: 1 hour. Cooking equipment: 2 saucepans, shallow open baking dish or casserole. Oven temperature: 180°C (350°F).

Chicken with Mustard Seed Sauce

Serves: 4

4 chicken fillets, skinless
½ cup tomato sauce
1 tsp tabasco sauce
2 tbsp seeded mustard
1 tbsp Worcestershire sauce
1 tbsp brown vinegar
1 clove garlic crushed

This is so easy to make and, once it's in the oven, you don't need to think about it again until you're ready to bring it to the table.

Method:

1. Arrange chicken in casserole.
2. Combine tomato sauce, tabasco sauce, mustard, Worcestershire sauce, vinegar and garlic.
3. Pour over chicken.
4. Cover and bake for 45 minutes. Alternatively, cover and microwave on 'medium' for 35 minutes.
5. Serve with cooked rice and hot vegetables or salad.

To store: cover and refrigerate for up to two days.

Nutrition data per serve: 749 kJ (179 cal), CHO 3 g, Protein 26 g, Fat 7 g.
Preparation time: 1 hour. Cooking equipment: casserole. Oven temperature: 180°C (350°F).

Five-spice Chicken

Serves: 4

¼ tsp Chinese five-spice powder
½ tsp chilli powder (or to taste)
1 tsp soy sauce
1 clove garlic, crushed
¾ cup low-fat natural yoghurt
4 chicken breasts, skinned

Method:

1. Fold five-spice powder, chilli powder, soy sauce and garlic gently into yoghurt.
2. Coat chicken breasts in yoghurt mixture and allow to stand at least 4 hours.
3. Place in shallow casserole, cover with lid or aluminium foil, and bake for an hour in a low to moderate oven or until tender, turning occasionally. Alternatively, microwave, covered, on 'medium' for 30 minutes or until tender, turning occasionally during the cooking process.

Note: this recipe is better cooked in a conventional oven than in the microwave.

Nutrition data per serve: 736 kJ (176 cal), CHO 4 g, Protein 28 g, Fat 6 g.
Preparation time: 1 ¼ hours, plus 4 hours marinating time. Cooking equipment: shallow casserole or baking dish. Oven temperature: 150°C (300°F).

Balinese Spiced Liver

Serves: 4

2 small onions, grated
1 clove garlic, crushed
¼ tsp ground turmeric
½ tsp brown sugar
pinch ground black pepper
1 tbsp soy sauce
1 bay leaf
1 tsp finely chopped chilli
1 tbsp peanut butter
juice of half a lemon
500 g (1 lb) chicken livers, sliced
1 cup coconut milk
garnish: 8 wedges of tomato, 12 wedges of cucumber

Liver should be prepared and eaten the same day. It's one of the richest sources of iron.

Method:

1. Mix all the ingredients, except the chicken livers and coconut milk, to make a soft paste. If the paste is too thick, add a little water. It should have the consistency of yoghurt.
2. In a saucepan, bring the paste to a gentle simmer and cook, stirring frequently, for 5 minutes.
3. Add the chicken livers and cook, stirring gently, until the livers change colour.
4. Add the coconut milk and slowly bring the mixture to the boil, stirring constantly. Then reduce heat and simmer for approximately 5 minutes until the mixture thickens.
5. Serve hot on a bed of boiled brown rice. Garnish with wedges of tomato and cucumber.

Nutrition data per serve: 1414 kJ (338 cal), CHO 7 g, Protein 31 g, Fat 21 g.

Preparation time: 30 minutes. Cooking equipment: medium-sized saucepan.

Chicken with Strawberry and Peppercorn Sauce

Serves: 4

2 tsp oil
4 chicken fillets
1 quantity Strawberry and Peppercorn Sauce (recipe, page 158)
garnish: 4 whole strawberries

Some unusual combinations don't quite make the mark, but this one is delicious and worthy of a special occasion. You don't have to go to the trouble of fanning the fillets or strawberries in the way we suggest, although this gives a professional touch; you can simply spoon the sauce over the cooked fillets and garnish them with halved strawberries.

Method:

1. Brush the frying pan with oil and heat over medium heat. Sauté the chicken fillets until cooked and golden brown. (You can microwave them on 'high' for 3 minutes but they will not brown.)

2. Prepare sauce as on page 158.
3. Slice whole strawberries leaving them joined at base. Fan out from top of strawberry (optional).
4. Slice fillets through and fan across each dinner plate.
5. Pour sauce over and garnish with fanned strawberries.

To vary: sliced turkey breast with Strawberry and Peppercorn Sauce makes a wonderful Christmas dinner.

Nutrition data per serve: 922 kJ (237 cal), CHO 7 g, Protein 30 g, Fat 8 g.
Preparation time: 15 minutes (including sauce). Chicken can be cooked while sauce is reducing. Cooking equipment: large frying pan.

Apricot Chicken

Serves: 4

2 cups canned apricots, packed solid
4 chicken breasts, skinned
1 large onion, chopped
coarsely ground black pepper, to taste
2 sage leaves, finely chopped or ½ tsp dried sage
1 sprig thyme, chopped
1 tbsp commercial fruit chutney
1 tbsp cornflour (cornstarch)
2 tbsp water
garnish: 4 apricot halves reserved from main quantity,
1 tbsp finely chopped chives or mint

Method:

1. Reserve four apricot halves for garnish. Purée remaining apricots in a food processor or blender or press through a sieve.
2. Arrange chicken fillets in a single layer in a casserole. Sprinkle over onion, pepper and herbs.
3. Combine chutney and apricot purée and pour over the chicken. Bake for 30 minutes.
4. Mix the cornflour (cornstarch) and water to a smooth paste.
5. Remove casserole from oven. Use a slotted spoon to lift out chicken breasts; cover and keep warm.
6. Drain the sauce from the casserole into a saucepan. Add the cornflour (cornstarch) paste to the sauce and heat, stirring constantly, until it thickens. Cook a further 2 minutes.
7. Arrange a chicken breast on each plate and spoon sauce over each one. Garnish with the reserved apricot halves and sprinkle over the chopped chives.

Nutrition data per serve: 805 kJ (192 cal), CHO 11 g, Protein 26 g, Fat 5 g.
Preparation time: 40 minutes. Cooking equipment: casserole, saucepan, food processor or blender.
Oven temperature: 180°C (350°F).

Chicken Tikka

Serves: 4

200 g (7 oz) low-fat natural yoghurt
juice 1 lemon
1 tsp finely chopped or minced ginger
1 tsp finely chopped or minced garlic
¼ tsp dried coriander
½ tsp powdered turmeric
2 tbsp chopped fresh mint
¼ tsp ground black pepper
¼ tsp garam masala
4 chicken breasts or thighs, skin removed

This is simple to make and superbly fragrant. All you need to add is plenty of carbohydrate-rich accompaniments and steamed vegetables or a crisp salad.

Method:

1. Combine yoghurt, lemon juice and flavourings in a bowl.
2. Add chicken and cover well with marinade. Cover and refrigerate for 2-3 hours.
3. Preheat oven.
4. Lift chicken from marinade. Place on baking dish. Cover with aluminium foil and bake for 30 minutes.
5. Remove foil, spoon remaining marinade over and bake until chicken is tender and lightly browned (½-1 hour).

Nutrition data per serve: 723 kJ (173 cal), CHO 4 g, Protein 27 g, Fat 6 g.

Preparation time: 2 hours. Cooking equipment: baking dish. Oven temperature: 200°C (400°F).

Saté Chicken

Serves: 4
(3 skewers each)

500 g (1 lb) chicken fillets
1 clove garlic, crushed
2 tbsp soy sauce
2 tbsp lemon juice
1 small onion, grated
1 tsp oil

A Malaysian recipe that makes a great alternative for the barbecue. Green prawns, pork, beef or lamb fillet are all delicious cooked with this marinade.

Method:

1. Cut chicken into small cubes.
2. Thread the chicken onto skewers. Arrange the skewers on a flat dish.
3. Combine remaining ingredients and brush over the chicken. Leave chicken to marinate for at least an hour, turning occasionally.
4. Grill or barbecue the saté chicken, turning frequently and basting from time to time with marinade.

5. Serve hot, accompanied by Peanut Sauce (recipe, page 155), Gado Gado (recipe, page 86) and brown rice.

To store: use on day of preparation. However, the dish may be made some hours ahead of time and kept, covered, in the refrigerator. You can freeze uncooked saté.

Nutrition data per serve: 708 kJ (169 cal), CHO 1 g, Protein 26 g, Fat 7 g.

Preparation time: 1½ hours (including marinading). Cooking equipment: 12 wooden skewers, (soak skewers in water for an hour before using to prevent burning) grill or barbecue.

Golden Chicken Risotto

Serves: 4

2 tbsp water
1 large onion, chopped
1 clove garlic, crushed
1½ cups uncooked brown rice
1½ litres (2½ pints) Chicken Stock (recipe, page 71) or 4 chicken stock cubes dissolved in 6 cups water
4 chicken breasts, skin removed, finely diced
1 tsp powdered turmeric
20 almonds, blanched and halved
3 tbsp raisins

There are two ways of preparing this dish — on top of the stove or in the oven. They are equally effective.

Method 1 — Preparing risotto on top of the stove:

1. In a large saucepan, heat the water to boiling, add the onion and cook until softened.
2. Add the garlic and cook for 2 minutes.
3. Add the rice and one quarter of the chicken stock. Bring to the boil. Reduce heat and simmer for 20 minutes, stirring occasionally and adding more stock, as necessary, to prevent sticking.
4. Add the diced chicken breasts, turmeric, almonds and raisins.
5. Continue simmering a further 20-25 minutes, adding remaining stock as necessary, until the rice is tender. There should be no liquid in the finished risotto.

Method 2 — Preparing risotto in a casserole:

1. Place all ingredients in a casserole.
2. Cover and cook in a preheated oven for 1 hour, or until rice has absorbed the stock and is tender.

Serve hot, accompanied by a green salad.

Nutrition data per serve: 2044 kJ (488 cal), CHO 65 g, Protein 32 g, Fat 11 g.

Preparation time: approximately 1 hour. Cooking equipment: saucepan, large saucepan or casserole with lid. Oven temperature: 180°C (350°F).

Chicken Enchiladas

Serves: 4

2 cups cooked, chopped chicken breast, skin removed

1 small onion, chopped finely

1 ripe avocado

juice 1/2 lemon

8-10 drops tabasco sauce or according to taste

1/4 tsp salt

1/4 tsp ground black pepper

4 small wholemeal pita bread or 2 sheets mountain bread

2 cups fresh tomato purée or commercial pasta sauce (meatless)

additional tabasco sauce to taste

1/2 cup low-fat block cheese, grated

Don't try storing the enchiladas, they will become soggy. You should serve them immediately they are heated through. Heat them in the oven, not in the microwave.

Method:

1. Combine chicken and onion in mixing bowl.
2. Peel avocado, remove stone. Mash flesh in a separate bowl with lemon juice.
3. Add tabasco sauce, salt and pepper and add to chicken mixture.
4. Mix well. Taste and adjust seasoning.
5. Split pocket breads in half so there are eight rounds (or cut each mountain bread into four).
6. Wrap each around one eighth of chicken mixture. Pack into casserole or baking dish.
7. Combine tomato purée with tabasco sauce, and pour tomato purée over chicken rolls.
8. Sprinkle with cheese.
9. Bake in a preheated oven until rolls are heated through and cheese has melted.

Nutrition data per serve: 2033 kJ (486 cal), CHO 26 g, Protein 39 g, Fat 25 g.

Preparation time: 1 hour. Cooking equipment: saucepan, shallow baking dish or casserole. Oven temperature: 200°C (400°F).

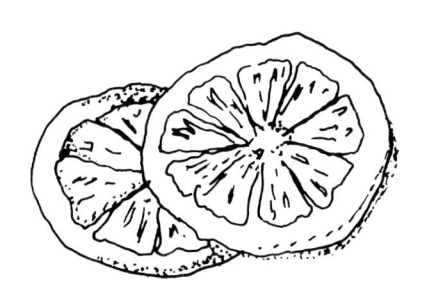

Chicken Soy

Serves: 4

4 spring onions (shallots), chopped
2 cloves garlic, crushed
2 tsp grated green ginger
1/3 cup soy sauce
3 tbsp dry sherry
4 chicken breasts, skinned
garnish: chopped parsley, chives or spring onions (shallots)

Try a garnish of three tablespoons of sesame seeds added before baking instead of the garnish suggested in the recipe.

Method:

1. Prepare the marinade. In a bowl, combine all the ingredients, except the chicken.
2. Arrange the chicken breasts in a baking dish. Pour over the marinade. Cover with plastic film and refrigerate for 2 hours, turning occasionally.
3. Bake them, uncovered, for 40 minutes, basting occasionally, or cover and microwave on 'medium' for 20-25 minutes.
4. Remove chicken from baking dish and arrange on a serving platter. Brush with pan juices. Sprinkle over with chopped parsley, chives or spring onions (shallots).

To store: cover and refrigerate for up to three days after cooking. Not recommended for freezing as the chicken dries out.

Nutrition data per serve: 685 kJ (164 cal), CHO 3 g, Protein 26, Fat 5 g.

Preparation time: 3 hours, including marinating time. Cooking equipment: baking dish. Oven temperature: 180°C (350°F).

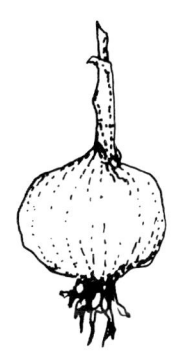

Drunken Rabbit Casserole

Serves: 4

800 g (1¾ lb) rabbit, jointed
1 tsp vinegar or lemon juice
1 medium onion, sliced
1 cup water
½ cup red wine
2 chicken stock cubes, crumbled
1 tbsp tomato paste
2 medium tomatoes, chopped
½ tsp dried oregano
6 spring onions (shallots), chopped
16 small button mushrooms or canned champignons
1 tbsp cornflour (cornstarch)
1 tbsp water

If rabbit is unavailable, you can use lean chicken instead. You'll need about 500 g (1 lb) of chicken breast.

Method:

1. Soak rabbit in cold water with a teaspoon of vinegar or lemon juice for 30 minutes. Discard water.
2. In a casserole, combine the rabbit, onion, 1 cup of water, wine, stock cubes, tomato paste, chopped tomatoes and oregano. Cover and bake for 1¼ hours, or microwave on 'medium' for 30-40 minutes.
3. Remove casserole from oven. Add the spring onions (shallots) and mushrooms and stir in. Cover, return to oven and bake a further 15 minutes or microwave on 'high' for 5 minutes.
4. Remove casserole from oven. Using a slotted spoon, lift the rabbit and vegetables onto a serving platter, cover and keep warm.
5. Pour the juices into a saucepan.
6. In a cup, stir the cornflour (cornstarch) and 1 tablespoon of water to make a smooth paste and add to the cooking juices. Bring to the boil, stirring constantly, until thickened. Reduce heat and simmer for 2 minutes.
7. Pour the sauce over the rabbit and vegetables and serve at once.

To store: cover and refrigerate for up to three days.

Nutrition data per serve: 997 kJ (238 cal), CHO 12 g, Protein 30 g, Fat 8 g.
Preparation time: 2¼ hours. Cooking equipment: casserole with lid, medium-sized saucepan. Oven temperature: 180°C (350°F).

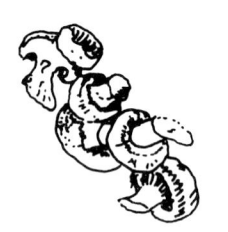

Sweet and Sour Rabbit with Prunes

Serves: 4

800 g (1¾ lb) rabbit, jointed
1 cup dry white wine
2 medium onions, skinned and sliced
1½ cups Chicken Stock (recipe, page 71) or 1½ cups water and 2 chicken stock cubes
1 bay leaf
1 tbsp redcurrant jelly
6-8 peppercorns, according to taste
8 whole prunes, stoned
¼ cup seedless raisins
1 tbsp malt vinegar
2 tbsp cornflour (cornstarch)
freshly milled black pepper
garnish: chopped parsley

Rabbit is low in fat and easy to prepare.

Method:

1. Marinate rabbit overnight in the wine and onions.
2. Discard the onions, place the rabbit and wine marinade in a flameproof casserole, and add the chicken stock, bay leaf, redcurrant jelly and peppercorns and bring to the boil. Turn down the heat.
3. Add the prunes and raisins, submerge them in the cooking liquid, cover the casserole tightly and bake slowly for about 1½ hours until the rabbit is tender and the prunes are plump.
4. Remove from oven, lift out the rabbit and remove the bones. Set meat aside and strain the cooking juices into a clean pan, retaining the prunes and raisins.
5. Blend cornflour (cornstarch) with vinegar to form a smooth paste, add to juices and boil for 1-2 minutes, stirring all the time until the sauce thickens. Arrange the rabbit, prunes and raisins in the casserole and pour the thickened juices over. Garnish with parsley.

Nutrition data per serve: 1152 kJ (275 cal), CHO 17 g, Protein 32 g, Fat 9 g.

Preparation time: 2 hours plus overnight soaking. Cooking equipment: large flameproof casserole with lid, medium saucepan. Oven temperature: 160°C (325°F).

Meatless Dishes

Jumping Bean Bake

Serves: 4 as a main course, 8 as a side dish

2 cups dried beans (any variety) or 4 cups canned and drained beans such as lima, bortolotti, kidney, soy, haricot
1 cup tomato purée
1/4 tsp cayenne pepper
2 gloves garlic, crushed
1 tsp dried oregano
1 bay leaf
500 g (1 lb) ripe tomatoes, sliced
2 medium onions, sliced
Topping:
1/2 cup fresh wholemeal breadcrumbs
4 tbsp grated, low-fat block cheese

For a thicker version of this dish, mash half the beans and leave the rest whole at Step 1 of the method described below.

Method:

1. Place dried beans in a saucepan, cover with water and soak overnight (note: do not soak the beans in an aluminium saucepan). Next day, drain the beans and rinse them thoroughly in cold water. Return them to the saucepan and cover with fresh water. Bring to boil, reduce heat and simmer, loosely covered, for 1 hour or until tender: or microwave on 'high' for 5 minutes, then 'medium-low' for 30 minutes or until tender. Drain beans, discarding water. If you are using canned beans, drain them and rinse them well.
2. In a bowl, combine the tomato purée, cayenne pepper, garlic and herbs.
3. Lightly grease the casserole, and place a layer of beans on the base, cover with a layer of tomatoes and then a layer of onions. Repeat the layers until all the ingredients are used.
4. Pour tomato mixture over, top with breadcrumbs and cheese.
5. Cover and bake for 1 hour, then remove cover and bake for another hour or until beans start to break apart. Alternatively, cover and microwave on 'medium' for 45 minutes, then remove the cover and microwave for another 30 minutes or until the beans start to break apart.
6. Serve immediately.

To store: cover and refrigerate for up to two days.

Nutrition data per serve (main meal): 1601 kJ (382 cal), CHO 55 g, Protein 29 g, Fat 4 g.
Preparation time: 2 1/4 hours after you have soaked dried beans overnight.
Cooking equipment: medium saucepan, deep casserole. Oven temperature: 180°C (350°F).

Foreground: simple lettuce salad, centre, Corn, Peas and Red Pepper with Curried Tuna and Rice Casserole. Top left, Fruit Crumble and Custard Sauce. Fresh pears at top right.

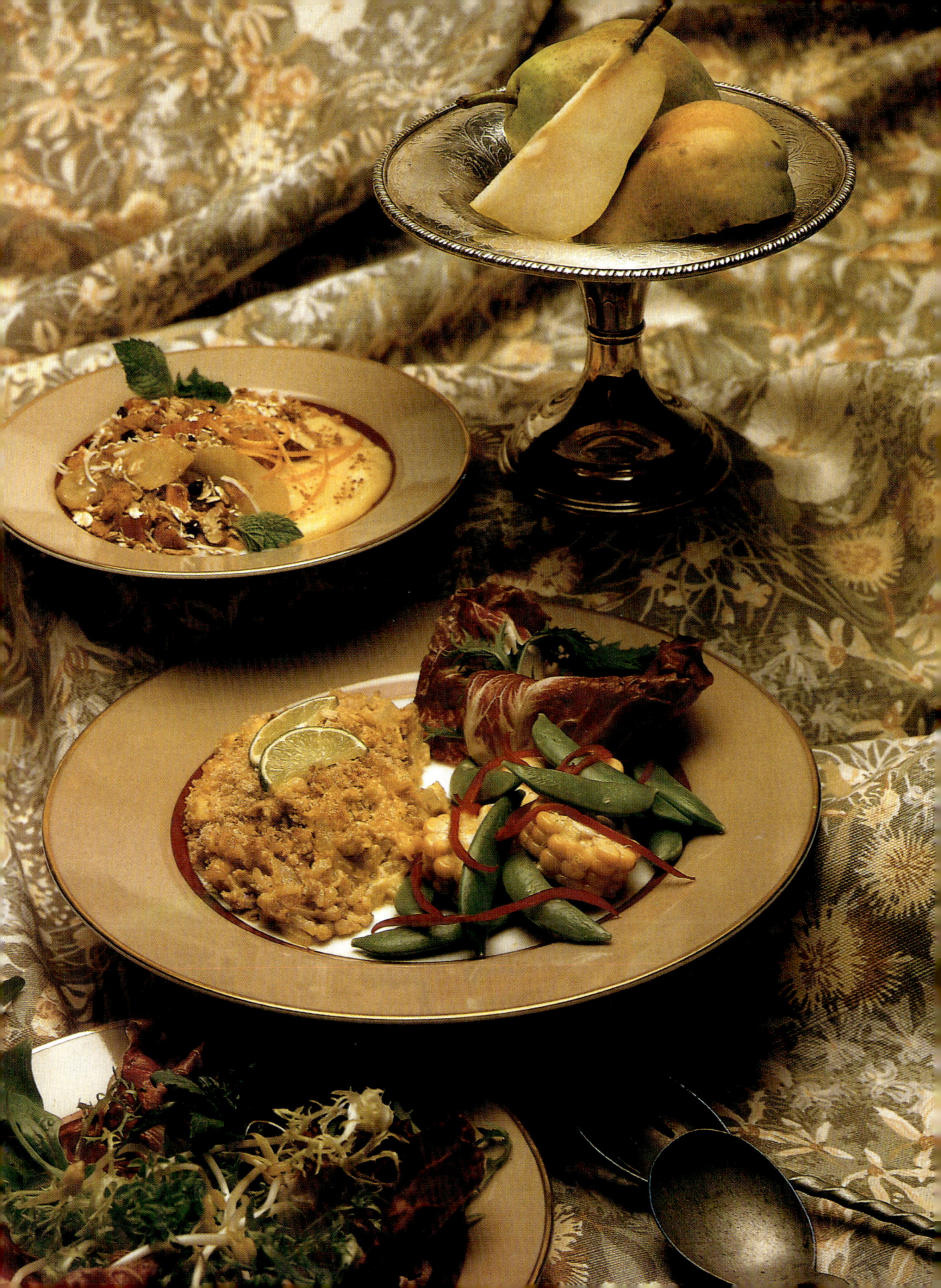

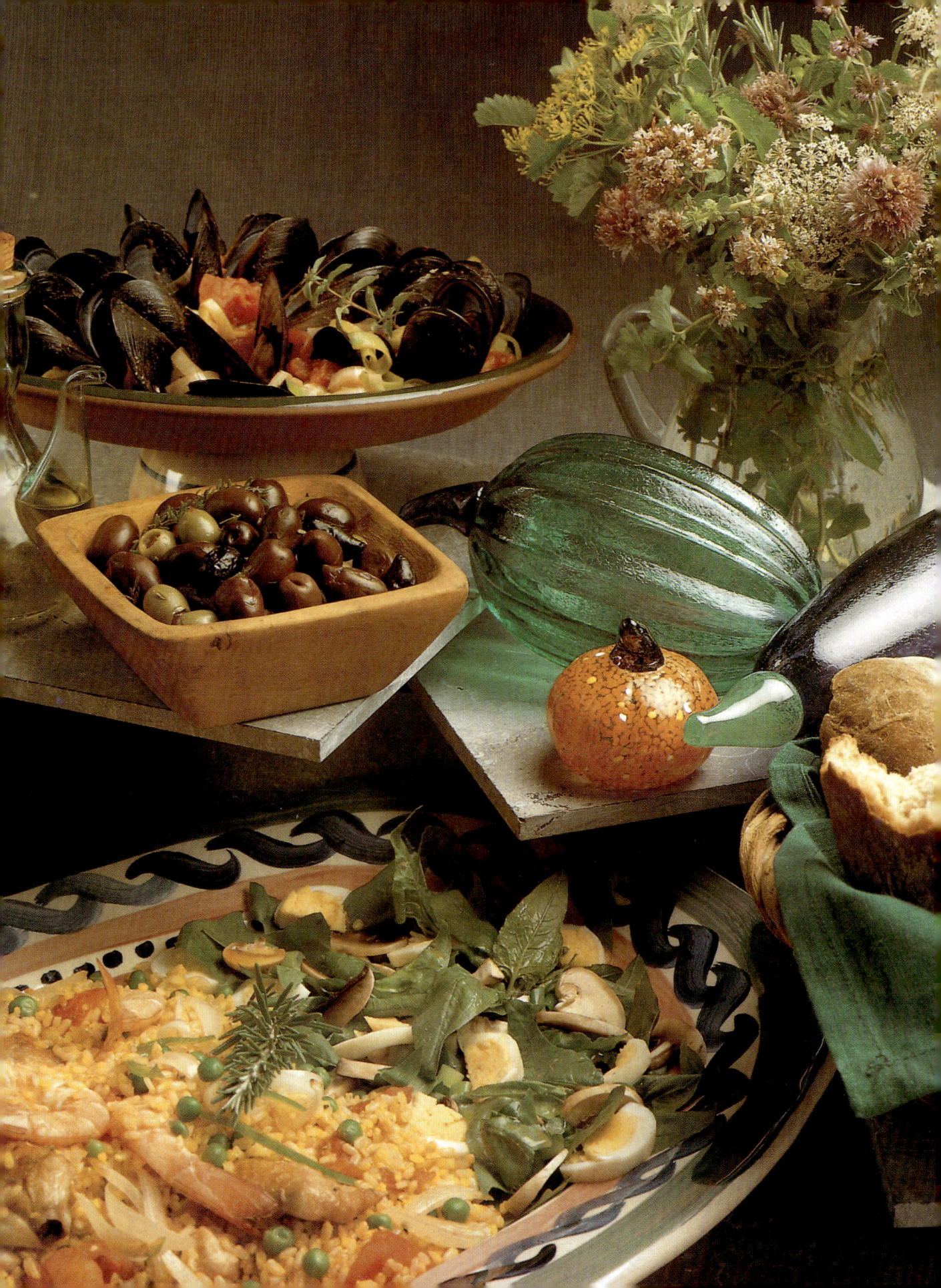

Vegetable Loaf

Serves: 6

2 tbsp water
2 medium onions, chopped
2 sticks celery, chopped
½ green capsicum (bell pepper), chopped
2 tsp curry powder
½ cup cooked potato, mashed
½ cup cooked pumpkin, mashed
1 cup ricotta cheese
1 cup coarsely ground cashew nuts
½ cup rolled oats
2 tbsp chopped parsley
1 tsp chopped fresh thyme or ½ tsp dried
garnish: 2 tbsp sesame seeds
For serving
1 quantity Cheese Sauce (recipe, page 155) or Fresh Vegetable Sauce (recipe, page 156)

This loaf is very high in fibre, and is delicious eaten hot or cold with one of the sauces we recommend.

Method:

1. In a frying pan, or in a bowl in the microwave, heat the water and sauté onions, celery, capsicum (bell pepper) and curry powder for 3 minutes.
2. In a bowl, combine the sautéed vegetables with the rest of the ingredients.
3. Line a loaf tin with foil and spray it with non-stick baking spray.
4. Sprinkle sesame seeds over base of tin, and then shake tin so that seeds adhere to sides as well.
5. Spoon vegetable mixture into the tin and press down firmly and neatly.
6. Bake for 40 minutes.
7. Remove from oven and leave to stand for 5 minutes before turning out. Turn onto serving dish and carefully remove foil.
8. Finally, grill on 'high' for 3-5 minutes or until the top is crisp and well browned.

To serve: cut loaf into thick slices, but do not separate them, then spoon hot sauce over it.

To store: cover and refrigerate for up to four days.

Nutrition data per serve : 1781 kJ (425 cal), CHO 25 g, Protein 29 g, Fat 24 g.

Preparation time: 1 hour plus preparation time for sauce. Cooking equipment: frying pan, loaf tin 20 cm x 10 cm (8 in × 4 in).
Oven temperature: 180°C (350°F), grill on 'high'.

Foreground: Paella accompanied by Spinach Valentino. Olives at centre and Mussels à la Grecque at the top.

Eat & Enjoy   Meatless Dishes

Vegetarian Lasagne

Serves: 4-6

Sauce:
oil
2 medium onions, peeled and chopped
3 large tomatoes, chopped
150 g (5 oz) tomato paste
2 cups water
1-2 tsp crushed or finely chopped garlic
1 tsp dried mixed herbs
¼ tsp each, black pepper and salt
750 g (26 oz) can three-bean mix or kidney beans

Layers:
250 g (8 oz) frozen spinach
9 sheets instant spinach or wholemeal lasagne noodles
½ cup each, cottage cheese and grated low-fat block cheese
2 tbsp grated parmesan cheese

This dish is even better if prepared the day before it is to be served, so that the flavour can fully develop. It freezes well, so prepare a few and store them in the freezer as a standby.

Method:

1. Wipe a frying pan with oil, heat it and sauté onions in frying pan until lightly browned, stirring to prevent burning.
2. Add tomatoes and cook for about 5 minutes until soft.
3. Add tomato paste and water and mix thoroughly.
4. Add seasonings.
5. Rinse and drain beans and add. Combine well.
6. Simmer gently, covered, until you are ready to assemble the lasagne. If sauce becomes too thick, add a little water.
7. Place spinach in saucepan. Cook very gently, uncovered, until it is fairly dry.

To assemble:

8. Spoon a thin layer of tomato and bean sauce over base of dish.
9. Arrange a layer of noodles on top.
10. Spoon on more sauce, sprinkle with half the low-fat cheese and 1 tbsp of parmesan.
11. Top with another layer of noodles and cover this with spinach, cottage cheese and the remaining parmesan.
12. Place the last layer of noodles over this, cover with the remaining sauce and, lastly, sprinkle with the remaining grated, low-fat cheese.
13. Cover with foil and bake for 30 minutes. Remove the foil, and bake for a further 30 minutes or until noodles are tender.

Nutrition data per serve (to serve 5): 1369 kJ (327 cal), CHO 42 g, Protein 25 g, Fat 6 g.

Preparation time: 2 hours. Cooking equipment: frying pan, small saucepan, square baking dish. Oven temperature: 180°C (350°F).

Cheese and Spinach Rolls

Serves: 4

1 bunch fresh spinach or 250 g (8 oz) packet frozen spinach
2 tbsp water
4 spring onions (shallots), chopped
1 cup ricotta cheese
1 cup cooked brown rice
2 tbsp lemon juice
pinch nutmeg
12 sheets filo pastry
2 tbsp skim milk

Serve these fragrant rolls with Cheese Sauce (recipe, page 155) spooned over them. Try adding 2 tbsp of pine nuts or chopped walnuts to the filling mixture.

Method:

1. Wash fresh spinach very thoroughly under cold, running water. Do not dry it. Chop roughly. Place wet, chopped spinach in a large saucepan. Cover and cook over high heat for about 10 minutes or until tender. Remove spinach from saucepan and drain well. Set aside to cool. (If you use frozen spinach, cook it uncovered in a saucepan over low heat until excess water has evaporated; set aside to cool.)
2. Bring water to the boil in a saucepan, add the spring onions (shallots) and cook until softened.
3. Combine onions with spinach, cheese, rice, lemon juice and nutmeg and blend well.
4. Fold a sheet of filo pastry in half widthwise. Brush lightly with milk.
5. Repeat with another two sheets of filo. Place them on top of the first, and brush milk between each sheet. You now have six layers of pastry.
6. Place a quarter of the filling along the edge of the pastry and roll up to encase the filling. Lift and tuck in the ends of the pastry before the last roll. This makes a neat parcel.
7. Place the completed roll, seal-side down, on a lightly greased baking tray.
8. Repeat Steps 4 to 7 to make four cheese and spinach rolls.
9. Brush each roll with milk. Bake for 15 minutes or until pastry is crisp and golden.

To store: cover and refrigerate for up to three days. Freezing: do not allow the rolls to brown too much during cooking as they will colour further when reheated. Freeze cooked rolls in suitable containers. Thaw completely before reheating.

Nutrition data per serve: 1139 kJ (272 cal), CHO 37 g, Protein 14 g, Fat 7 g.
Preparation time: 45 minutes. Cooking equipment: medium saucepan, baking tray.
Oven temperature: 200°C (400°F).

Tibetan Pie

Serves: 6

1 quantity Wholemeal Pastry (recipe, page 190)
Filling:
6 medium potatoes, washed but not peeled, cut into large pieces
500 g (1 lb) frozen spinach
1 large onion, chopped
4 tbsp chopped fresh mixed herbs (mint, thyme, parsley, oregano, marjoram)
½ tsp coarsely ground black pepper
1 tsp salt (optional)
¼ tsp nutmeg
1 tsp curry powder
2 tsp margarine

Keep pastry cool in the refrigerator while preparing the filling; this prevents the pastry from becoming soggy when you add hot filling.

Method:

1. Cook spinach in saucepan until excess water has evaporated. The spinach should be fairly dry.
2. Boil potatoes until tender. Drain and mash potatoes roughly so that some pieces remain.
3. Add spinach, onion, herbs, spices and margarine.
4. Cut pastry into two (⅔ and ⅓).
5. Roll out larger piece to cover base and sides of pie dish.
6. Spoon filling onto pastry, brush pastry edge with a little water.
7. Roll out smaller piece of pastry. Place on top of filling. Pierce the top of the pastry with a fork.
8. Trim the pastry to size and pinch the edges of pastry together.
9. Bake for approximately 45 minutes or until lightly browned.

Nutrition data per serve: 1776 kJ (424 cal), CHO 50 g, Protein 12 g, Fat 19 g.

Preparation time: 1½ hours. Cooking equipment: 2 saucepans, pie dish. Oven temperature: 200°C (400°F)

Spanish Omelette

Serves: 5

2 tsp margarine
3 medium potatoes, diced but not peeled
1 large onion, chopped
6 mushrooms, chopped
1 green capsicum (bell pepper), chopped
½ cup cooked vegetables (corn, peas, carrots)
½ stick celery, chopped

Delicious cold or hot, and is a great way of using up leftover cooked and uncooked vegetables. It also makes a nutritious school or office lunch.

Method:

1. Melt margarine in frying pan over medium-high heat.
2. Add potato and onion. Cover and cook over low heat for approximately 15 minutes until potatoes are tender.
3. Add mushrooms, capsicum (bell pepper), cooked vegetables and celery and cook a further 5 minutes.
4. Beat eggs with seasonings and water.

5 eggs
¼ tsp black pepper
¼ tsp ground nutmeg
1 tsp dried mixed herbs
pinch salt (optional)
2 tsp chopped parsley
few drops tabasco sauce or pinch cayenne pepper
¼ cup water

5. Pour over vegetables in frying pan, cover, and cook over low heat until almost set. Do not allow bottom to burn.
6. Preheat grill to medium, and slide omelette under the grill to complete cooking.
7. Loosen omelette and turn onto warm plate.
8. Cut into wedges to serve.

To store: cover and refrigerate for up to two days.

Nutrition data per serve: 688 kJ (164 cal), CHO 16 g, Protein 10 g, Fat 7 g.

Preparation time: 45 minutes. Cooking equipment: large heavy-based frying pan.

Vegetable Curry

Serves: 4

500 g (1 lb) mixed vegetables
2 tsp oil
1 onion, sliced
1 tsp ground turmeric
½ tsp ground cumin
2 cm (¾ in) piece green ginger, chopped
2 cloves garlic, chopped
1 or 2 fresh hot chillies (optional) or chilli powder to taste
1 cup water
1 cup coconut milk
1 tbsp lemon juice

Using a variety of vegetables makes this an economical dish based on whatever vegetables are in season. Beans, cabbage, broccoli, cauliflower, pumpkin, sweet potatoes, spinach, potatoes, peas, carrots, eggplant (aubergine) and zucchini are ideal.

Method:

1. Trim vegetables and cut into pieces.
2. Heat oil until very hot in wok or large frying pan.
3. Add onion and spices and toss until onion is golden brown.
4. Add the rest of the vegetables and stir-fry for 2-3 minutes.
5. Add 1 cup of water and cook 6-8 minutes, uncovered, or until vegetables are tender.
6. Add coconut milk and bring to boil.
7. Remove from heat. Add lemon juice.
8. Serve with brown rice.

Nutrition data per serve: 657 kJ (157 cal), CHO 8 g, Protein 4 g, Fat 12 g.

Preparation time: 45 minutes. Cooking equipment: wok or frying pan.

Semolina Gnocchi with Tomato and Basil Sauce

Serves: 4

1½ cups skim or low-fat milk
½ tsp ground nutmeg
1 cup semolina
2 eggs
small amount of plain flour
1 cup of Tomato and Basil Sauce (recipe, page 156) or 1 cup commercial tomato-based pasta sauce

Gnocchi are best served fresh, but you can refrigerate them for up to three days and then reheat them by dropping them in boiling water. Or prepare the gnocchi to Step 5 then freeze, completing the preparations from Step 6 when you need to serve them.

Method:

1. Place milk and nutmeg in medium saucepan and bring to boil. Remove from heat and quickly stir in semolina.
2. Return to heat and stir for 1 minute.
3. Add eggs and work into a smooth dough.
4. Break off small, even-sized pieces about the size of a walnut, roll into balls and toss in a little flour.
5. Half fill a large saucepan with water and bring to the boil.
6. Drop gnocchi into boiling water and cook for about 5 minutes (gnocchi will rise to the top of the water as they cook).
7. Drain. Toss in sauce and serve immediately.

Nutrition data per serve: *1076 kJ (257 cal), CHO 38 g, Protein 12 g, Fat 6 g.*
Preparation time: 30 minutes plus preparation time for sauce. Cooking equipment: medium saucepan, a large saucepan.

Potato Gnocchi

Serves: 4

500 g (1 lb) potatoes, peeled, cooked and mashed
½ cup plain flour
½ cup wholemeal flour
1 quantity Fresh Vegetable Sauce (recipe, page 156)
4 tbsp grated, low-fat block cheese

You can also prepare gnocchi to Step 3 and then freeze them. When you are ready to use the gnocchi, drop them into boiling water and follow the recipe from Step 4.

Method:

1. Half fill saucepan with water and place on stove to boil. A little salt may be added to the cooking water if desired.
2. Mix potato with both flours, then turn onto a floured board and knead gently until smooth.
3. Divide mixture into four, and roll each into a sausage about 2 cm (¾ in) in diameter. Cut lengths into 2 cm (¾ in) pieces and drop into boiling water.

4. Boil gently for 8-10 minutes until gnocchi are light and cooked (gnocchi will rise to surface of the water as they cook).
5. Use a slotted spoon to remove onto a serving dish.
6. Toss in sauce, sprinkle with cheese and serve immediately.

To vary: sprinkle with 4 tbsp chopped lean ham, or use Tomato and Basil Sauce (recipe, page 156) instead of Fresh Vegetable Sauce.

Nutrition data per serve: 1222 kJ (292 cal), CHO 50 g, Protein 14 g, Fat 4 g.

Preparation time: 15 minutes plus preparation time for sauce. Cooking equipment: large saucepan.

Pita Pizza

Serves: 4

4 small wholemeal pita breads
1 cup Tomato and Basil Sauce (recipe, page 156) or 1 cup commercial pasta sauce
3 large tomatoes, sliced
1 medium green capsicum (bell pepper), deseeded and sliced
1 cup sliced mushrooms
1 medium onion, peeled and sliced
8 tbsp grated, low-fat block cheese
oil
Options: 16 black olives, chopped
1 zucchini, sliced

The beauty of this recipe is that by using pita bread as the pizza base, you can put the whole dish together very quickly. These pizzas freeze well, making them an ideal snack or light meal.

Method:

1. Spread pita breads with sauce. Arrange the vegetables evenly over the top and sprinkle with grated cheese.
2. Place on a lightly oiled baking tray. Bake for 20 minutes or until cheese melts and begins to brown.
3. Serve pita pizzas straight from the oven, accompanied by a Tossed Salad (recipe, page 153).

To store: prepare pizzas in advance up to Step 2, wrap in plastic film or slide into big freezer bags and freeze until needed; then place the frozen pizzas on a baking tray and bake for 25 minutes.

Nutrition data per serve: 1404 kJ (335 cal), CHO 42 g, Protein 17 g, Fat 11 g.

Preparation time: 30 minutes plus preparation time for sauce. Cooking equipment: large saucepan, baking tray. Oven temperature: 180°C (350°F).

Mexicale Pie with Cornmeal Dumplings

Serves: 4

2 tsp oil

1 finely chopped onion

2 cloves garlic, crushed

1 green capsicum (bell pepper), diced

2 tbsp tomato paste

440 g (14 oz) can whole tomatoes

440 g (14 oz) can corn kernels, drained

780 g (26 oz) can kidney beans, drained

½ tsp allspice

1 tsp chilli powder or to taste

1 bay leaf

2 tsp Worcestershire sauce

½ cup water

cornmeal dumpling mixture:

1 cup each, wholemeal self-raising flour and yellow cornmeal (polenta)

¾ cup low-fat milk

2 eggs, lightly beaten

1 cup low-fat block cheese

2 tbsp chopped chives

The dumplings give this already nutritious and flavoursome dish an extra carbohydrate punch. Experiment with the flavourings according to your taste for spicy food. We have suggested canned vegetables and beans to make the dish quick to prepare.

Method:

1. Heat oil in the saucepan over medium heat and then sauté onion, garlic and capsicum (bell pepper) for approximately 3 minutes until just tender.
2. Add tomato paste, vegetables, spices, bay leaf, Worcestershire sauce and water.
3. Boil uncovered for 15 minutes, then remove bay leaf.
4. Transfer bean mixture to baking dish or casserole.
5. Make the dumplings by combining all the ingredients. Drop spoonfuls of dumpling mixture on top of the bean mixture.
6. Bake, uncovered, for 10 minutes, then reduce heat to 180°C (350°F) and bake for another 30 minutes. Serve hot.

Nutrition data per serve: 3160 kJ (755 cal), CHO 99 g, Protein 48 g, Fat 17 g.

Preparation time: 1¼ hours. Cooking equipment: saucepan, shallow baking dish or casserole. Oven temperature: 200°C (400°F) then 180°C (350°).

Spinach Fettuccine

Serves: 4

2 bunches fresh spinach or 500 g (1 lb) frozen spinach
250 g (8 oz) spinach fettuccine
2 tbsp pine nuts
1 tbsp water
1 small onion, finely chopped
½ clove garlic, crushed
1 tsp chopped fresh basil, or ½ tsp dried basil
coarsely ground black pepper to taste
250 g (8 oz) ricotta cheese

This dish should always be eaten freshly prepared.

Method:

1. Trim away the roots and woody ends of stems of fresh spinach. Rinse spinach thoroughly in cold, running water, but do not dry. Heat a large saucepan. Put the spinach into the saucepan, cover and cook over medium-high heat for 5-8 minutes or until tender. Remove from heat and drain in a colander. Set aside.
   If you are using frozen spinach, place it in a saucepan and thaw over low-medium heat. Remove from heat, drain well and squeeze to remove excess liquid. Set aside.
2. Fill a large saucepan two-thirds with water, and bring to a rapid boil. Add the fettuccine and boil for 10-12 minutes or until it is *al dente* (tender, but firm to bite). Drain.
3. Meanwhile, in a dry frying pan, brown the pine nuts over medium heat, stirring constantly to ensure even colouring and prevent burning. Remove from frying pan and set aside.
4. Return frying pan to the heat. Add the tablespoon of water, onion, garlic, basil and pepper. Cook over low heat until the onion is translucent.
5. In a large saucepan, combine the cooked spinach, pine nuts, ricotta cheese and the onion mixture. Add the fettuccine, use two forks to gently lift and turn mixture to combine well.
6. Serve hot.

Nutrition data per serve: 1573 kJ (376 cal), CHO 47 g, Protein 20 g, Fat 11 g.
Preparation time: 30 minutes. Cooking equipment: 2 large saucepans, frying pan.

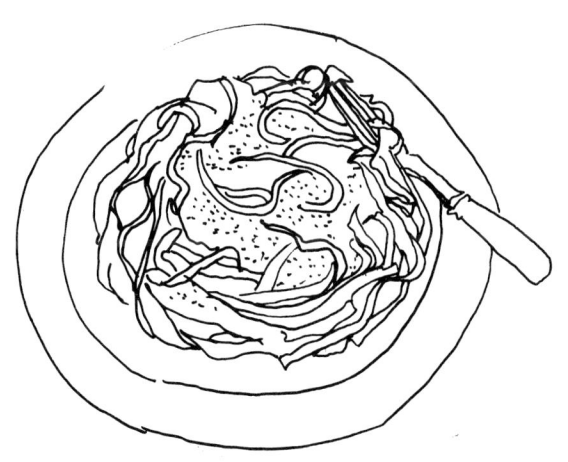

Claytons Quiche

Serves: 4

4 eggs
1 cup skim milk
1 cup full-cream natural yoghurt
2 tbsp wholemeal flour
1 cup ricotta cheese
½ cup chopped spring onions (shallots)
120 g (4 oz) mushrooms, sliced
1 medium tomato, diced
oil
330 g (11 oz) can asparagus, drained

This quiche makes its own crust. It is quick and easy to make, and is delicious hot or cold served with crusty bread and green salad. Will keep in the refrigerate for up to three days.

Method:

1. Beat together eggs, milk, yoghurt and flour.
2. Add cheese, spring onions (shallots), mushrooms and tomato.
3. Pour into a lightly oiled flan dish.
4. Arrange asparagus on top.
5. Bake for 30-35 minutes or until quiche is set and lightly browned.

Nutrition data per serve: 1146 kJ (274 cal), CHO 15 g, Protein 23 g, Fat 14 g.

Preparation time: 1 hour. Cooking equipment: flan dish. Oven temperature: 180°C (350°F).

Bubble and Squeak

Serves: 4

2 tsp oil
1 medium onion, finely sliced
4 cups cooked, mixed vegetables (e.g.: potato, cabbage, pumpkin, carrot, cauliflower, broccoli, beans, peas, spinach and zucchini)
black pepper to taste

Method:

1. In a frying pan, heat the oil. Add the onion and sauté gently until lightly browned.
2. Add mixed vegetables and pepper. Use a metal spatula to lift and turn mixture until well combined. Then press down vegetables to make a flat cake in the frying pan.
3. Cook over medium heat for 5 minutes, or until the bottom of the 'cake' is well browned.
4. Cut into wedges in the frying pan. Serve brown side up.

Nutrition data per serve: 445 kJ (106 cal), CHO 13 g, Protein 7 g, Fat 3 g.

Preparation time: starting with pre-cooked vegetables, 10 minutes. Cooking equipment: large frying pan.

Vegetable Side Dishes

Vegetables have tended to become a neglected part of the meal. Yet with a little imagination they can be a feature.

Try mixing vegetables in different combinations, and experiment with adding fresh or dried herbs and seasonings. Nutmeg, curry powder, onion, chives, tomato, garlic, wine or a sprinkle of toasted sesame seeds or almonds provide a delicious flavour boost. The following ideas may help get you started **on a new appreciation of the versatility of vegetables**. All the suggestions are for four people.

Braised Onion

Place 1 cup of water and a chicken stock cube in a saucepan and bring to the boil. Add 4 small, peeled and sliced onions and simmer them for about 8 minutes until they are tender. Lift out the onions and set them aside, add 2 tablespoons of dry white wine to the stock and boil the liquid until it is reduced to about 3 tablespoons. Add the onions, heat through and serve them garnished with chopped chives or parsley.

Braised Lettuce

Wash an iceberg lettuce and remove any stalks or damaged outside leaves. Cut the lettuce into wedges. Bring 2 cups of chicken stock to the boil, drop in the lettuce wedges and simmer them for 15-20 seconds. Lift them out and, if desired, serve them garnished with finely sliced spring onion (shallot) tops.

Lemon Broccoli

Wash 1 large head of broccoli, removing the woody stem. Cut the broccoli into even florets and steam or boil them for 4-6 minutes until they are tender but still crisp. Drain the broccoli. Alternatively, microwave them on 'high' for 4 minutes. Finally, toss them in a mixture of lemon juice, the rind of 1 lemon and 2 teaspoons of toasted sesame seeds.

Spinach and Spring Onions (Shallots)

Wash a bunch of fresh spinach under running water, remove all trace of dirt. Destalk. Chop the spinach finely and place it in a saucepan with a bunch of chopped spring onions (shallots), 2 tablespoons of finely chopped parsley, a pinch of nutmeg and 2 tablespoons of water. Cover and cook for 5-6 minutes. Alternatively cover and microwave it on 'high' for 4-5 minutes. Serve immediately.

Diced Parsleyed Potatoes

Scrub 4 medium potatoes and cut them into 2 cm (3/4 in) cubes. Drop them into boiling water and simmer them gently for 8-10 minutes until tender. Drain. Alternatively, microwave them on 'high' for 7-8 minutes. Finally, sprinkle them with parsley and toss gently.

Snow Peas and Asparagus

Cut 20 asparagus spears to about the length of the snow peas, discarding the woody ends. Plunge the asparagus (from which you have removed the stalks) into boiling water for 2 minutes until the asparagus spears are tender. Add 20 snow peas, return to the boil and then drain. Make sure that the vegetables don't overcook. Place them on a serving dish and sprinkle them with toasted sesame seeds or almond slivers.

This recipe can be varied by replacing the asparagus with whole green beans or celery strips. These vegetables are microwaved on 'high' for 2-3 minutes.

Succotash (peas, capsicum (bell peppers) and corn)

Boil or steam 1-1½ cups each of frozen peas and corn kernels for 4-5 minutes. Drain. Alternatively cover and microwave them on 'high', for 4 minutes. Then add a diced red capsicum (bell pepper), mix thoroughly, season with freshly ground black pepper and serve.

Pumpkin and Mushrooms

Peel and seed 4 medium pieces of pumpkin and slice each into pieces about 1 cm (½ in) thick. Place them in a saucepan with 6 sliced mushrooms, a cup of unsweetened tomato juice, a crushed clove of garlic and ground black pepper. Simmer gently for about 15 minutes until the vegetables are tender or, alternatively, place all the ingredients in a microwave dish, cover and microwave on 'high' for 8 minutes.

Zucchini and Carrot Rings

Trim and slice thickly 4 medium zucchini and cut half a medium carrot into thin rings. Heat 2 teaspoons of oil in a large saucepan, add the carrots and cook, tossing them constantly, for 2 minutes. Add the zucchini and cook, tossing them constantly, for a further 2 minutes. Add ½ cup of water, cover and cook for about 5 minutes until tender. Drain and season with ground black pepper and chopped parsley.

Leek and Apple

Wash and slice a large leek. Peel and slice a large cooking apple. Heat a tablespoon of water in a saucepan, add the leek and apple and toss them to mix. Cover and cook over low heat for approximately 8 minutes until tender. Alternatively, microwave the leek, apple and water on 'high' for 5 minutes.

Zucchini Creole

Peel and quarter a medium onion, cut half a medium green capsicum (bell pepper) into strips. Place them and 2 tablespoons of water in a saucepan and cook for 2 minutes. Add 4 quartered tomatoes, 4 zucchini cut into wedges, 12 pitted black olives and ½ teaspoon of chopped fresh basil (¼ tsp dried), cover and simmer gently for 10 minutes.

Scalloped Potatoes

Serves: 4

6 medium potatoes, scrubbed
1 cup skim milk
¼ tsp coarsely ground black pepper
1 tsp chopped parsley
¼ tsp dried mixed herbs

This is an ideal dish, high in complex carbohydrate. It is wonderfully satisfying just as it is, but lends itself equally to tempting variations. We have given two options, but you can experiment with your own. Although scalloped potatoes are usually eaten hot, they can also be served cold.

Method:

1. Slice potatoes finely. Arrange in overlapping rows or circles in a shallow baking dish.
2. Pour over skim milk and sprinkle with pepper, parsley and herbs.
3. Bake for 30 minutes or until potatoes are tender and slightly browned on top, or microwave, covered, on 'high' for 20 minutes.

As an accompaniment: serve hot with meat, fish or chicken.

To vary: omit mixed herbs and sprinkle with sweet paprika to taste, or after the potatoes have been in the oven for 25 minutes, remove them and sprinkle them with grated, low-fat block cheese, and then return to the oven for 5 minutes or until the topping is golden and bubbling.

To store: Store covered in refrigerator for up to 2 days.

Nutrition data per serve: 566 kJ (135 cal), CHO 26 g, Protein 7 g, Fat trace.
Preparation time: 35 minutes. Cooking equipment: shallow, medium-sized baking dish. Oven temperature: 180°C (350°F).

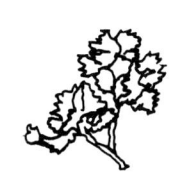

Jacket Potatoes

Serves: 4 as an accompaniment; 2 as a light meal

---

4 medium-sized potatoes

Method:

1. Wash potatoes well, do not peel. Prick several times with a fork or skewer. For a crispy skin: do not cover. For a softer skin: wrap potatoes in foil.
2. Bake the potatoes for 45-60 minutes or until tender when tested with a skewer.

Alternatively, wash and with a fork prick potatoes and cook uncovered in the microwave on 'high' for 12 minutes, turning them over halfway through cooking.

Serve plain or try some of the following delicious fillings, or a combination of your own.

Preparation time: 70 minutes. Cooking equipment: baking tray. Oven temperature: 180°C (350°F).

Cheese and pastrami	Slice tops off potatoes and scoop out flesh, leaving 4 firm shells. Cut 2 small, thin slices of pastrami into fine strips and mix with 60 g (2 oz) grated low-fat block cheese, the flesh from potatoes and 2 tbsp low-fat milk. Add a little ground black pepper, spoon back into potato shells and reheat in oven for about 5-10 minutes.
Cottage cheese (or yoghurt) and chives	Split open tops of potatoes and place ½ tbsp cottage cheese or low-fat natural yoghurt in each. Sprinkle with chopped chives and serve immediately.
Tomato and onion	Sauté 1 finely chopped onion in a little water, add 1 medium chopped tomato, ½ tsp chopped fresh basil or oregano and a pinch of ground black pepper. Mix with flesh from potatoes, spoon into potato shells and reheat in oven for about 5-10 minutes.
Spicy yoghurt	Combine the flesh of potatoes with 2 tbsp low-fat natural yoghurt and a pinch each of ground ginger, cinnamon and cloves. Spoon back into potato shells and reheat in oven for about 5-10 minutes.

Duchess Potatoes

Serves: 4

4 medium-sized old potatoes
1 egg
1 tsp margarine
white pepper to taste
pinch salt (optional)
garnish: nutmeg

Method:

1. Wash, peel and rinse potatoes.
2. Cut into even-sized pieces.
3. Place in small quantity of boiling water and cook until soft (about 20 minutes) or microwave on 'high' covered until soft.
4. Drain and mash potatoes.
5. Beat egg and put aside 1 tsp for glazing.
6. Beat potatoes, margarine and egg together until fluffy.
7. Season with pepper (and salt, if desired).
8. Pipe onto an oven tray to form cone shapes.
9. Glaze with remaining egg.
10. Sprinkle with nutmeg.
11. Brown in oven for 10 minutes.

Nutrition data per serve: 425 kJ (102 cal), CHO 15 g, Protein 5 g, Fat 2 g.

Preparation time: 30-40 minutes. Cooking equipment: saucepan, oven tray, piping bag and nozzles. Oven temperature: 200°C (400°F).

Curried Brussels Sprouts with Almonds

Serves: 4

20 brussels sprouts, with stems trimmed and slit
1 tsp margarine
2 tbsp blanched, slivered almonds
2 tsp water
1 small onion, finely diced
1 tsp Curry Powder (recipe, page 164)

Method:

1. Drop the brussels sprouts into a saucepan containing 2 cm (¾ in) boiling water and boil rapidly for about 5 minutes, or until cooked, but still firm.
2. Dry the saucepan and return to heat.
3. Melt margarine in saucepan, add almonds and toss until lightly brown, remove from pan.
4. Add 2 tsp water, onion, and curry powder and stir until onions are lightly cooked.
5. Return sprouts and almonds to saucepan, toss to mix and serve.

Nutrition data per serve: 312 kJ (75 cal), CHO 3 g, Protein 5 g, Fat 5 g.

Preparation time: 10 minutes. Cooking equipment: saucepan.

Dry Curry of Potato, Eggplant (Aubergine) and Pea

Serves: 4

1 tbsp ghee or unsalted butter or margarine
1½ tsp panch phora
1 large onion, finely chopped
2 tbsp mint, chopped
1 tsp fresh ginger, finely chopped
¼ tsp ground chilli
1 tsp ground turmeric
500 g (1 lb) potatoes, peeled and diced
500 g (1 lb) eggplant (aubergine), diced
250 g (8 oz) frozen or fresh green peas
3 tbsp hot water
1 tsp garam masala
1 tbsp lemon juice
salt to taste (optional)

Method:

1. Heat the ghee and fry the panch phora until seeds start to brown.
2. Add onion and fry until soft.
3. Add mint, ginger, chilli and turmeric and stir.
4. Add vegetables and water, mix well and cover.
5. Reduce to a low heat and cook for 20 minutes shaking pan occasionally to toss vegetables and to prevent them burning.
6. Sprinkle with garam masala, lemon juice and salt, cover and cook for a further 10 minutes.
7. Serve hot.

Ideal to accompany Indian Lamb in Spinach Sauce (recipe, page 107).

Nutrition data per serve: 734 kJ (175 cal), CHO 24 g, Protein 8 g, Fat 5 g.

Preparation time: 45 minutes. Cooking equipment: 1 large saucepan with fitted lid.

Note: Spices used in Indian curries are usually available in large supermarkets and are also readily available in Asian grocery shops.

Panch phora can be purchased pre-mixed. It is a mixture of five different types of seed used whole:

1 quantity fenugreek seeds and fennel seeds to double quantity black mustard seeds, cumin seeds and black cumin seeds.

Garam masala can be purchased pre-mixed. It is a mixture of ground spices which may vary in type and amount: e.g. coriander, cumin, cardamom, cinnamon, cloves and nutmeg.

...otato Patties

meal plings?

Serves: 4

orange
...oes (yams)
... pepper to taste
¼ tsp ground cardamom
¼ tsp ground turmeric
½ tsp finely chopped or minced ginger
2 tsp chopped parsley
2 tbsp chopped chives
⅓ cup sesame seeds

Method:

1. Peel sweet potatoes (yams) and cut into pieces.
2. Place in saucepan with 1-2 cups water (or steam or microwave) and the cardamom, and cook until tender.
3. Drain, remove the cardamom and mash the potatoes.
4. Add the other spices, ginger, parsley and chives. Then cover and cool (approximately 1 hour).
5. Shape into patties (four large or eight small).
6. Coat with sesame seeds.
7. Place on baking tray, bake for approximately 30 minutes or until sesame seeds are toasted and patties are heated through.

To vary: replace sesame seed with wheatgerm.

Nutrition data per serve: 699 kJ (167 cal), CHO 29 g, Protein 7 g, Fat 2 g.
Preparation time: 2 hours. Cooking equipment: medium saucepan, baking tray. Oven temperature: 200°C (400°F).

Mushroom and Pecan Rice

Serves: 4

½ cup Chicken Stock (recipe, page 71) or 1 stock cube in ½ cup water
6 mushrooms, sliced
4 spring onions (shallots), cut into 1 cm (½ in) lengths
2 tbsp chopped pecan nuts
2 cups cooked brown or basmati rice

This filling dish has the complex carbohydrate we need. It's also wonderfully quick to prepare. Try using walnuts or pine nuts instead of pecan nuts. If you decide to use onions in place of the spring onions (shallots), then add a tablespoon of chopped parsley as well.

Method:

1. Heat chicken stock in large pan or wok.
2. Cook mushrooms and onions in stock for 3-4 minutes.
3. Add nuts and rice and toss while heating through.

Serve hot or chill and serve cold.

Nutrition data per serve: 767 kJ (183 cal), CHO 31 g, Protein 4 g, Fat 5 g.
Preparation time: 15 minutes. Cooking equipment: large pan or wok.

Eat & Enjoy   Vegetable Side Dishes

Mushroom Stroganoff

Serves: 4

2 tbsp water
2 onions, sliced
1 red or green capsicum (bell pepper), diced
16-20 medium-sized button mushrooms, sliced
3 spring onions (shallots), chopped
2 tsp paprika
1 cup low-fat, natural yoghurt
garnish: 3 tbsp chopped parsley

Serve this dish with brown rice, noodles or beancurd. Or use it as a topping for jacket potatoes. It makes an excellent piquant sauce for grilled meats or fillets of chicken and fish.

Method:

1. In the frying pan, bring the water to a simmer and add the onion, red or green capsicum (bell pepper) and the mushrooms. Simmer gently for 5 minutes.
2. Add spring onions (shallots) and paprika and simmer gently, stirring occasionally, for a further 5 minutes, or microwave for a further 2 minutes on 'high'. Remove from heat.
3. Place yoghurt in a bowl, gradually fold in mushroom mixture. Do not reheat as yoghurt will curdle. Garnish.

Nutrition data per serve: 249 kJ (59 cal), CHO 8 g, Protein 6 g, Fat 1 g.

Preparation time: 15 minutes. Cooking equipment: frying pan.

Curried Potatoes and Cauliflower

Serves: 4

1-2 tsp Curry Powder, according to taste (recipe, page 164)
2 medium potatoes, scrubbed and diced
½ cauliflower, separated into florets
1 bay leaf
1 cup boiling water
garnish: 2 tsp chopped parsley

The flavour of curried food improves with standing, so this dish can be prepared 24 hours in advance and stored, well covered, in the refrigerator. Reheat before serving.

Method:

1. Dry fry the curry powder in the base of large saucepan for 1 minute, stirring constantly.
2. Add all the other ingredients.
3. Cover saucepan and leave to simmer gently for 20 minutes, or until vegetables are tender and the water absorbed. Remove bay leaf. Serve hot, garnished with parsley.

Nutrition data per serve: 218 kJ (52 cal), CHO 9 g, Protein 3 g, Fat trace.

Preparation time: 30 minutes. Cooking equipment: saucepan.

Zucchini and Tomato Bake

Serves: 4

2 tsp margarine or oil
1 round of mountain bread
2 medium zucchini cut in half, crossways, and then into strips
3 tomatoes, sliced
4 spring onions (shallots), chopped
2 tsp fresh herbs, chopped, or 1 tsp dried mixed
pinch salt (optional)
pinch pepper
½ medium onion, sliced very finely
2 tbsp sesame seeds
Sauce:
1 tbsp tahina paste
juice ½ lemon
¼ tsp finely chopped or minced fresh ginger
¼ tsp prepared mustard
water to blend to a thin paste

Method:

1. Spread margarine or oil over casserole.
2. Place bread in this. Push into corners without breaking it, and leave excess hanging out.
3. Place half of the zucchini in the bottom.
4. Cover with the sliced tomato.
5. Sprinkle spring onions (shallots), herbs, salt and pepper over.
6. Place the remainder of the zucchini over this, then finely sliced onion.
7. Blend sauce ingredients.
8. Pour mixture over vegetables.
9. Sprinkle with sesame seeds.
10. Fold edges of bread in around the edge of the casserole to form a crust around the edge.
11. Bake for 40-45 minutes or until the bread is brown and crusty, and the zucchini is tender.

Nutrition data per serve: 633 kJ (151 cal), CHO 21 g, Protein 7 g, Fat 4 g.

Preparation time: 15 minutes. Cooking equipment: shallow casserole. Oven temperature: 200°C (400°F).

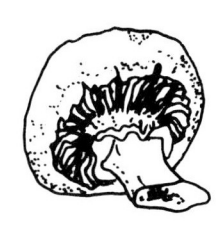

Spiced Rice with Peas

Serves: 4

1 tbsp polyunsaturated vegetable oil
1 tsp fresh ginger, finely chopped
½ fresh chilli, finely chopped or ½ tsp minced chilli paste
¼ tsp black mustard seeds
¼ tsp cumin seeds
2 curry leaves
3 cups water
1 cup basmati rice
100 g (3 oz) frozen peas
2 tsp each of fresh coriander, mint, and basil, chopped
¼ tsp ground saffron
salt to taste

Method:

1. Heat oil in pan, add ginger, chilli, mustard and cumin seeds and cook, stirring, for 1 minute.
2. Add water, bring to boil and add all other ingredients, cover and return to boil.
3. Reduce heat and simmer for 15 minutes or until rice is tender.

Suitable to accompany Mogul Lamb (recipe, page 108).

Nutrition data per serve: 985 kJ (235 cal), CHO 42 g, Protein 5 g, Fat 5 g.

Preparation time: 25 minutes. Cooking equipment: 1 medium saucepan.

Eggplant Neapolitan

Serves: 4

1 large or 2 small eggplant (aubergine), peeled and thinly sliced
4 large tomatoes, sliced
2 onions, sliced
½ tsp mixed dried herbs
ground black pepper to taste
1 clove garlic, crushed
1 cup tomato juice or purée

Method:

1. Layer vegetables in casserole.
2. Sprinkle with herbs, pepper and garlic and pour tomato juice or purée over.
3. Bake uncovered for 45 minutes.

Nutrition data per serve: 258 kJ (62 cal), CHO 11 g, Protein 4 g, Fat trace.

Preparation time: 1 hour. Cooking equipment: deep casserole. Oven temperature: 180°C (350°F).

Vegetables en Brochette

Serves: 4

16 cherry tomatoes
16 pearl onions, peeled (or small pieces of onion)
16 button mushrooms, stalks trimmed
1 medium green capsicum (bell pepper), cut into 2 cm (¾ in) squares
2 tbsp lemon juice
2 tsp soy sauce

When you prepare this dish, allow two tomatoes, two onions, two mushrooms and two or three pieces of green capsicum (bell pepper) per skewer. Serve it with brown rice or on a bed of cracked wheat and you have the basis of a delectable meal.

Method:

1. Thread vegetables evenly along skewers, leaving about 2.5 cm (1 in) of skewer free at each end.
2. Mix lemon juice and soy sauce, and brush mixture over vegetables.
3. Grill for about 5 minutes on each side until vegetables are tender. During grilling, brush with lemon juice and soy sauce mixture at intervals to prevent drying.
4. Serve hot.

Nutrition data per serve: 139 kJ (33 cal), CHO 5 g, Protein 3 g, Fat trace.

Preparation time: 20 minutes. Cooking equipment: eight 18 cm (7 in) skewers.

Orange-glazed Parsnips

Serves: 4

2 medium parsnips, scrubbed and sliced
1 tsp grated orange rind
½ cup orange juice
2 tsp margarine

Carrots cooked this way are splendid, too.

Method:

1. Drop parsnips into boiling water and cook until almost tender (about 5 minutes), or microwave, covered, with 2 tablespoons of water for 3 minutes until almost tender.
2. Drain, add orange rind, juice and margarine to parsnips.
3. Bring to boil and cook for a further 3 minutes, or microwave, covered, on 'high' for a further 2 minutes.
4. Lift out parsnips and keep warm.
5. Return saucepan to heat and simmer orange sauce to allow it to reduce and thicken.
6. Once sauce has thickened pour over parsnips, reheat quickly and serve.

Nutrition data per serve: 246 kJ (59 cal), CHO 8 g, Protein 1 g, Fat 2 g (carrot variation: 185 kJ (44 cal), CHO 6 g, Protein 1 g, Fat 2 g).
Preparation time: 15 minutes. Cooking equipment: saucepan. Oven temperature: 180°C (350°F).

Vegeballs

Serves: 4

2 tsp margarine
12 small white or pearl onions
12 button mushrooms (or canned champignons)
12 cherry tomatoes
coarsely ground black pepper

Method:

1. Melt margarine in pan or wok.
2. Add onions and toss gently for 3-4 minutes until beginning to soften.
3. Add mushrooms and continue tossing until they darken evenly.
4. Add tomatoes and very gently toss until they are heated through.
5. Sprinkle with black pepper.

To vary: substitute small white or pearl onions with 2 cm (¾ in) lengths of spring onion (shallots).

Nutrition data per serve: 155 kJ (37 cal), CHO 3 g, Protein 2 g, Fat 2 g.
Preparation time: 15 minute. Cooking equipment: large frying pan or wok.

Sweet and Sour Red Cabbage

Serves: 4

500 g (1 lb) red cabbage, shredded
1 onion, chopped
1 cooking apple, peeled, cored and chopped
1 clove garlic, crushed
1 tbsp vinegar
1 tsp caraway seeds
pepper to taste
3 tbsp water

This makes a wonderful companion dish to rice, noodles or potato. Add a small portion of grilled fish or meat and you have the basis for a well-balanced meal.

Method:

1. Place cabbage, onion, apple, garlic, vinegar, caraway seeds, and pepper in a saucepan or microwave-proof bowl.
2. Cook over a low heat for 5 minutes, stirring frequently or microwave on 'high' for 3 minutes.
3. Add the water, bring to the boil and simmer for 10 minutes or microwave on 'high' for a further 5 minutes.
4. Serve by arranging the cabbage on a hot serving dish, sprinkled with parsley.

Nutrition data per serve: 204 kJ (49 cal), CHO 8 g, Protein 3 g, Fat trace.
Preparation time: 30 minutes. Cooking equipment: saucepan.

Crunchy Peasant Rice

Serves: 4

½ bunch spinach or silverbeet
1 tbsp water
1 small onion, chopped
2 cups cooked brown rice
3 tsp soy sauce
2 tbsp chopped brazil nuts

Almonds or pine nuts are as good in this dish as the brazil nuts.

Method:

1. Wash spinach or silverbeet thoroughly, and cook without any additional water in the saucepan or microwave about 2 minutes.
2. Drain well and chop coarsely.
3. Heat large pan, add 1 tbsp water and sauté onion until transparent.
4. Toss all ingredients lightly together in pan until heated through.

To store: cover and refrigerate for up to three days. Reheat before serving or serve cold.

Nutrition data per serve: 945 kJ (226 cal), CHO 37 g, Protein 6 g, Fat 6 g.
Preparation time: 10 minutes. Cooking equipment: large saucepan or microwave dish, large frying pan.

Vegetables Julienne

Serves: 4

1 small zucchini
2 medium carrots
8 french beans
1 stick celery
½ green capsicum (bell pepper)
4 spring onions (shallots)
1½ cups water
1 chicken stock cube

Prepare the vegetables neatly using a small sharp knife. Cook them quickly and serve them right away.

Method:

1. Trim top from zucchini. Cut in half, across, then in half lengthways and, finally, into julienne strips.
2. Peel carrots, cut as for zucchini. Top and tail beans. Cut each in half, across, then in half lengthways.
3. Cut celery into lengths, then into strips. Cut capsicum (bell pepper) into strips, removing any pith and seeds.
4. Trim spring onions (shallots), cut into lengths, then each length in half.
5. Add water and stock cube to saucepan, bring to boil.
6. Add carrots, cook 2-3 minutes, then beans, celery and zucchini and cook a further minute.
7. Lastly, add capsicum (bell pepper) and spring onions (shallots) and cook a further minute.
8. Drain, then gently lift vegetables from water, using tongs or a slotted spoon to avoid breaking strips.

Nutrition data per serve: 146 kJ (35 cal), CHO 6 g, Protein 2 g, Fat trace.
Preparation time: 20 minutes. Cooking equipment: saucepan.

Hot Shredded Beets

Serves: 4

2 medium beetroot
2 tsp margarine
6 spring onions (shallots), chopped
¼ tsp black pepper
pinch salt (optional)

Beetroot has a sweetness that adds contrast to a meal.

Method:

1. Top and tail beets, peel and grate.
2. Heat margarine in a frying pan over medium-high heat, and add beetroot, spring onions (shallots), black pepper and salt.
3. Sauté gently, turning from time to time, for about 10 minutes or until cooked through.

Nutrition data per serve: 222 kJ (53 cal), CHO 7 g, Protein 2 g, Fat 2 g.
Preparation time: 20 minutes. Cooking equipment: frying pan.
Foreground: Turkey with Strawberry and Peppercorn Sauce with Orange glazed Parsnips, steamed snowpeas and asparagus. Front left Gazpacho. Then Christmas Pudding smothered in Brandy Sauce, and beribboned Christmas Cake.

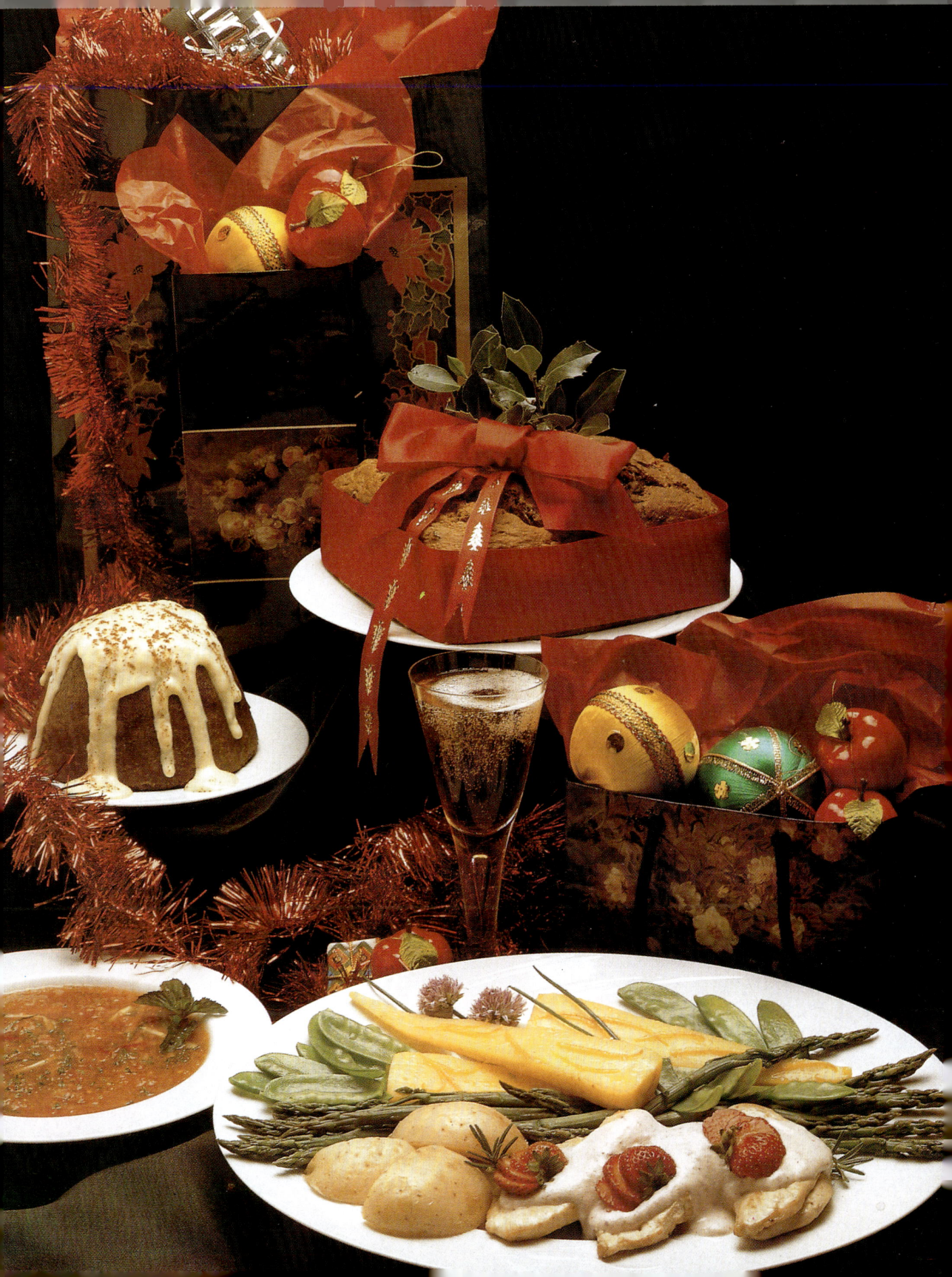

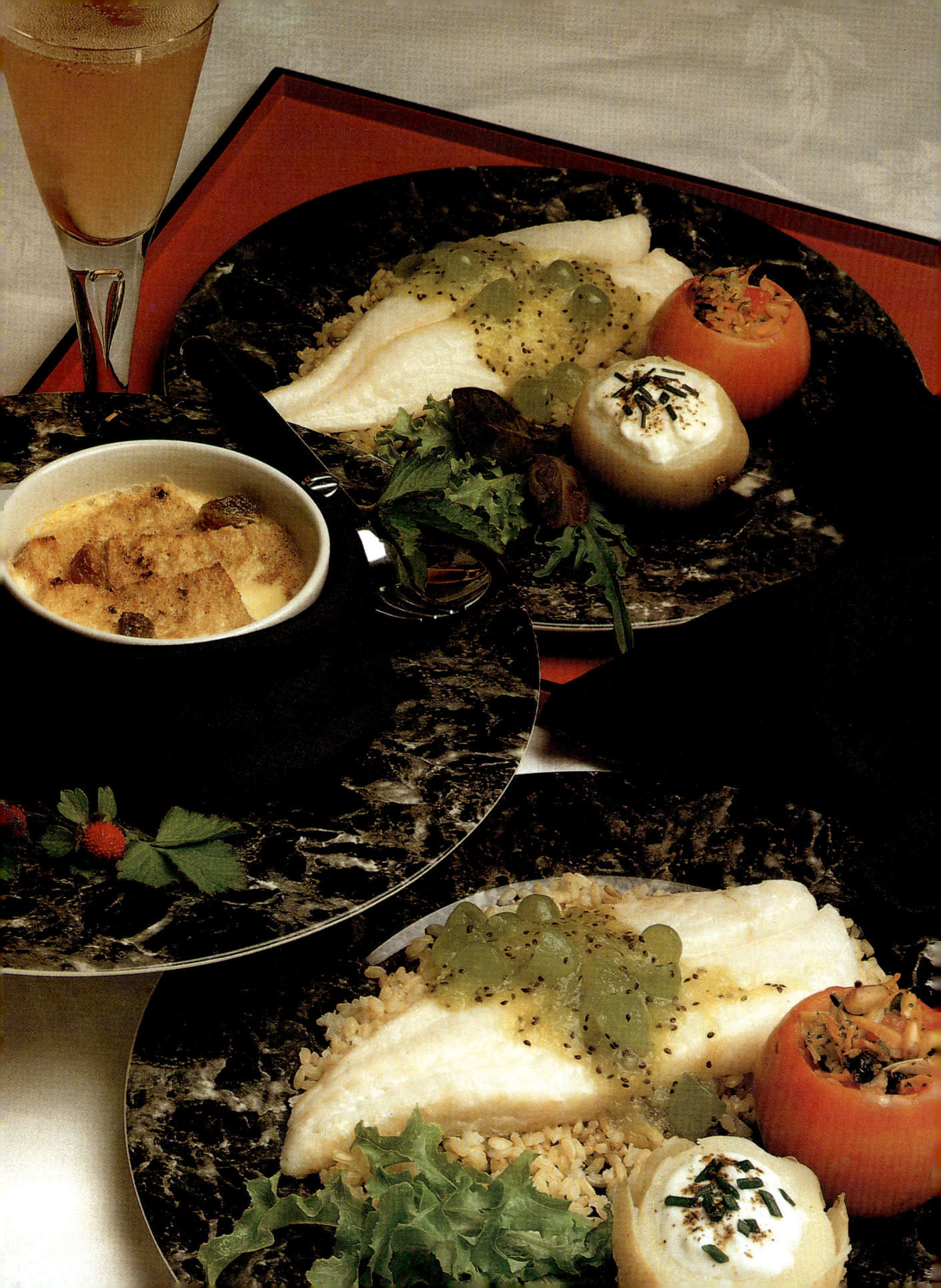

Stir-fried Vegetables

Serves 4

½ Chinese cabbage or ⅛ green cabbage
1 tsp oil
1 small white onion, quartered
1 tsp minced ginger
¾ cup broccoli florets
1 small carrot, sliced finely
10-12 snow peas
¾ cup bean shoots
½ green capsicum (bell pepper), diced
100 g (3 oz) mushrooms, sliced
½ cup water
1 stock cube
1 tbsp soy sauce

Stir-fried vegetables should be crisp and fresh-coloured — the result of swift cooking over high heat.

Method

1. Prepare the Chinese cabbage by cutting off the woody ends of stalks. Discard. Cut the stalks into 2 cm (1 in) lengths and shred the leaves. Cut the cabbage leaves into shreds about 5cm (2 in) long.
2. Place wok or heavy frying pan over high heat. Coat thinly with the oil. When very hot add fresh ginger and onion. Stir-fry for 2-3 minutes.
3. Add remaining vegetables, stir-fry for 2-3 minutes more.
4. Dissolve the stock cube in water, then add to vegetables.
5. Turn the heat down, add the soy sauce and combine with the vegetables. Cover the wok or pan, and simmer vegetables for 3-4 minutes. Serve hot.

Nutrition data per serve: 172 kJ (41 cal), CHO 6 g, Protein 4 g, Fat 1 g.

Preparation time: 20 minutes. Cooking equipment: wok or heavy frying pan.

Cracked Wheat

Serves: 4

1½ cups burghul (cracked wheat)
1½ cups Chicken Stock (recipe, page 72)

In line with the new way to eat, carbohydrate should be central to the meal. Cracked wheat prepared this way is quick and easy. Use it to build a meal just as you would with, say, brown rice or wholemeal noodles.

Method:

1. Wash wheat under cold running water.
2. Place in saucepan, pour chicken stock over. Simmer for 10-15 minutes until tender.

Nutrition data per serve: 593 kJ (139 cal), CHO 26 g, Protein 6 g, Fat 1 g.
Preparation time: 15 minutes. Cooking equipment: saucepan.

Foreground: Jacket Potato with Yoghurt and Chives beside Stuffed Tomato served with Fish and Green Champagne Sauce. Centre left, Bread and Butter Pudding with Custard.

Salads

All the salad ideas we give here are simple, but show you that with a little inspiration a salad can add something special to a meal. All these recipes will serve four.

Asparagus and Green Bean Salad

Trim 8 spears of fresh asparagus and cut them into 7 cm (3 in) lengths. Top, tail and halve 12 green beans. Boil, steam or microwave them until just tender, then drop them into icy water to cool them quickly. This helps retain their crispness and colour. Drain. Wash and dry a mignonette lettuce, tear it into pieces and line a salad bowl. Combine the asparagus, beans and 16 cherry tomatoes and place them in the salad bowl. Pour over ¼ cup of Italian Dressing (recipe, page 160) and sprinkle 2 tablespoons of toasted sesame seeds over.

Ginger Carrots

Slice 2 medium carrots into long strips with a potato peeler. Add a little peeled and finely chopped fresh ginger and then pour ½ cup of vinegar over. Refrigerate for 2 hours before serving. You can add thinly sliced cucumber if you like.

Tomato and Onion

Slice 3 firm, ripe tomatoes and a white onion. Pour ½ cup of brown vinegar over. Add freshly ground black pepper. Refrigerate for at least ½ hour before serving.

Orange and Cucumber Salad

Peel and slice 2 oranges, removing all pith. Slice ½ cucumber and a small onion. Break the onion into separate rings. Mix and sprinkle them with a tablespoon of chopped parsley and, finally, pour over one quantity of Creamy Orange Dressing (recipe, page 161). Chill well before serving.

Mushroom Salad

Slice 10 medium mushrooms into a bowl. Add a cup of beanshoots, ½ cup each of celery and red capsicum (bell pepper), cut into matchsticks, and 2 chopped spring onions. Toss with ½ quantity of Orange and Soy Dressing (recipe, page 160) or Herbed Tomato Dressing (recipe, page 161) and chill well.

Avocado, Spinach and Tofu Salad

Wash a bunch of spinach, remove the stalks and tear the leaves into bite-size pieces. Place spinach in a bowl and add a sliced medium avocado, 8 pitted and quartered black olives and 250 g (8 oz) firm tofu (soyabean curd) cut into small cubes. Make a dressing of 2 teaspoons of olive oil, 1 tablespoon lemon juice and a crushed clove of garlic, pour it over the salad and toss lightly. Chill.

Broccoli, Beanshoots and Snowpeas with Lemon

Blanch 2 cups broccoli florets by cooking them in boiling water or steaming them for 3 minutes. Plunge quickly under cold water to cool . Steam 12-15 (150 g/5 oz) snowpeas for 1-2 minutes and cool quickly under cold water. Rinse 1 cup of beanshoots and combine them with the broccoli and snowpeas in a bowl. Pour over a dressing made of 2 tablespoons of lemon juice, ½ teaspoon of coarsely ground black pepper and 2 teaspoons of oil. Serve chilled.

Fruity Noodle Salad

Serves: 4

2½ cups cooked noodles
½ cup sultanas
1 stick celery, diced
3 spring onions (shallots), chopped
1 green apple, cored and diced
4 dried apricots, chopped
4 dried peaches, chopped
⅓ cup pine nuts
Dressing:
½ cup orange juice
1 clove garlic, crushed
1 tsp minced ginger
1 tsp lemon juice
1 sachet Equal™ or other sweetener equivalent to 2 tsp sugar

Method:

1. Combine all ingredients, except the pine nuts, in salad bowl.
2. Toast pine nuts until golden brown in a moderate oven for 5-8 minutes. Cool and then add to other ingredients.
3. Combine the dressing ingredients in a screw top jar, shake well and pour over salad.
4. Toss salad, cover and refrigerate for several hours before serving.

To store: keep in airtight container in refrigerator for up to three days.

Nutrition data per serve: 1368 kJ (327 cal), CHO 56 g, Protein 9 g, Fat 8 g.

Preparation time: 15 minutes. Cooking equipment: baking tray.
Oven temperature: 180°C (350°F).

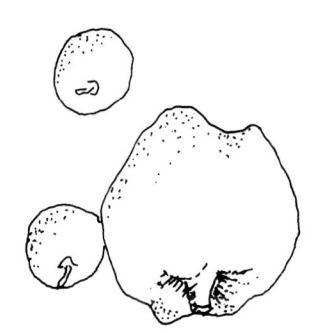

Curried Pasta Salad

Serves: 4

1½ cups uncooked shell noodles
½ cup diced celery
4 spring onions (shallots), chopped
2 tbsp sultanas
½ green capsicum (bell pepper), diced
2 tbsp chopped parsley
½ cup corn kernels
Dressing:
½ quantity Curry Dressing (recipe, page 161)

Method:

1. Cook noodles in boiling water for 10-12 minutes until *al dente* (tender), drain and then run cold water over to cool them.
2. Combine noodles, celery, spring onions (shallots), sultanas, capsicum (bell pepper), parsley and corn.
3. Toss in curry dressing.
4. Refrigerate for 1 hour before serving.

To store: keep in airtight container in refrigerator and store for up to two days.

Nutrition data per serve: 556 kJ (133 cal), CHO 26 g, Protein 5 g, Fat 1 g.

Preparation time: 1¼ hours. Cooking equipment: saucepan.

Spinach Valentino

Serves: 4

1 bunch spinach
4 mushrooms, sliced
2 spring onions (shallots), sliced
2 eggs, hardboiled
1 quantity Orange and Soy Dressing (recipe, page 160)

Method:

1. Wash spinach thoroughly, and shake gently to remove excess water. Remove the stalks and tear into bite-size pieces.
2. Combine spinach, mushrooms, spring onions (shallots) and sliced eggs and toss in dressing.
3. Chill before serving.

Nutrition data per serve: 266 kJ (63 cal), CHO 2 g, Protein 5 g, Fat 4 g.

Preparation time: 5 minutes.

New Potato Salad

Serves: 4

16 small new potatoes
2-3 tbsp fresh mint, chopped
2 tbsp chopped fresh chives or 2 tbsp chopped spring onion (shallots)
200 g (7 oz) low-fat natural yoghurt
½ tsp minced green ginger
½ tsp minced garlic
½ tsp prepared mild mustard
1 tsp lemon juice

Method:

1. Scrub potatoes if necessary, but do not peel.
2. Boil, steam or microwave the potatoes until tender. Drain and cool.
3. Place in serving bowl and add mint and chives or spring onions (shallots).
4. In a small mixing bowl combine yoghurt, ginger, garlic, mustard and lemon juice. Mix well.
5. Pour over potatoes. Mix well. Cover and refrigerate until ready to serve.

Nutrition data per serve: 343 kJ (82 cal), CHO 14 g, Protein 5 g, Fat 1 g.

Preparation time: 2¾ hours including cooling time.
Cooking equipment: medium saucepan.

Tabbouleh

Serves: 4

½ cup burghul (cracked wheat)
2 large ripe tomatoes, skinned and finely chopped
1 small onion, finely chopped
1 cup chopped parsley
ground black pepper
2 tsp olive oil
2 tbsp lemon juice
1 tbsp finely chopped mint

Method:

1. Place burghul in a deep bowl, cover with boiling water and allow to stand for 2 hours.
2. Drain well by squeezing in a clean muslin cloth or tea towel, and return to bowl.
3. Add the tomatoes, onion, parsley, pepper, oil, lemon juice and mint.
4. Combine well and chill for 1 hour before serving.

Nutrition data per serve: 470 kJ (112 cal), CHO 17 g, Protein 4 g, Fat 3 g.

Preparation time: soaking burghul 2 hours, preparation 15 minutes, chilling time 1 hour.

Curried Sweet Potato and Banana Salad

Serves: 4

3 medium orange sweet potatoes (yams), peeled
2 medium bananas
1 tbsp lemon juice
2 spring onions (shallots), chopped
1 quantity Curry Dressing (recipe, page 161)

Method:

1. Cut the sweet potato into 2 cm (¾ in) cubes.
2. Place in a large saucepan and barely cover with cold water. Bring to the boil, reduce heat and simmer for about 10-12 minutes, or until potato is cooked through, but still holds it shape. Alternatively, microwave on 'high' for 5-6 minutes.
3. Meanwhile, slice banana and toss in lemon juice.
4. Drain the cooked potato and allow to cool.
5. In a salad bowl place the potato, banana, spring onions (shallots) and dressing and toss gently to combine.

Nutrition data per serve: 524 kJ (125 cal), CHO 26 g, Protein 4 g, Fat 1 g.
Preparation time: 20 minutes. Cooking equipment: large saucepan.

Tangy Potato Salad

Serves: 4

3 medium potatoes
4 spring onions (shallots), chopped
3 eggs, hardboiled and sliced
½ cup low-fat natural yoghurt
½ tsp black pepper coarsely ground
2 tsp Curry Powder (recipe, page 164)
4 lettuce cups

This salad is best when made in advance; the flavour develops during refrigeration.

Method:

1. Peel potatoes.
2. Cook until slightly soft, but do not overcook as potato will not hold its shape. Drain.
3. Cut potato into cubes and mix with spring onion.
4. Add eggs.
5. Combine yoghurt, pepper and curry powder. Spoon over the potato mixture and toss gently.
6. Store in airtight container in refrigerator until required.
7. Serve in lettuce cups.

To store: cover and refrigerate for up to two days.

Nutrition data per serve: 550 kJ (131 cal), CHO 14 g, Protein 9 g, Fat 4 g.
Preparation time: 30 minutes. Cooking equipment: saucepan.

Coleslaw

Serves: 4

¼ medium cabbage, finely shredded
1 small onion, grated
1 small green capsicum (bell pepper), chopped
1 stick celery, chopped
⅓ cup grated carrot
ground black pepper
½ quantity Creamy Yoghurt Dressing (recipe, page 160)

Once you have added the dressing, coleslaw should not be stored. However, you can prepare the vegetables in advance and store them in the refrigerator. Add the dressing just before serving.

Method:

Toss all ingredients in a large bowl, chill until ready to serve.

To vary: add ⅓ cup chopped pineapple and 2 tablespoons of sultanas. Subsitute commercial low-oil coleslaw dressing for Creamy Yoghurt Dressing.

To store: cover and refrigerate for no more than a day.

Nutrition data per serve: 122 kJ (29 cal), CHO 5 g, Protein 2 g, Fat trace.

Preparation time: 10 minutes.

Broad Bean and Smoked Salmon Salad

Serves: 4

250 g (8 oz) broad beans, frozen or fresh
85 g (3 oz) smoked salmon, thinly sliced
12 cherry tomatoes
1 small white onion, thinly sliced
2 tbsp lemon juice
2 tsp olive oil
2 tsp capers, drained
2 tsp chopped fresh parsley

Method:

1. Cook broad beans until soft, but still retain their shape.
2. Combine broad beans, smoked salmon, cherry tomatoes and white onion in a bowl.
3. Blend all the other ingredients in a screw top jar and pour over the salad.
4. Chill and serve.

Nutrition data per serve: 414 kJ (99 cal), CHO 3 g, Protein 10 g, Fat 4 g.

Preparation time: 20 minutes. Cooking equipment: saucepan.

Fettuccine Salmon Salad

Serves: 4

4 cups water
250 g (8 oz) fresh spinach fettuccine
6 spring onions (shallots)
½ stick celery
½ capsicum (bell pepper)
1 tomato
½ zucchini
½ avocado
200 g (7 oz) can red salmon
1 cup grated carrot
Dressing:
2 tbsp chopped mint
juice ½ lemon
juice 1 orange
2 tsp olive oil
2 tsp soy sauce

Method:

1. Heat water until boiling.
2. Add fettuccine and cook until *al dente* (tender).
3. Drain, rinse and cool.
4. Chop spring onions (shallots), celery, capsicum (bell pepper) and tomato.
5. Cut zucchini into fine strips.
6. Peel avocado, discard stone, chop roughly.
7. Drain salmon, remove bones and skin.
8. Combine pasta with all other ingredients and mix gently.
9. Mix dressing ingredients and pour over. Serve.

Nutrition data per serve: 1189 kJ (284 cal), CHO 25 g, Protein 16 g, Fat 13 g.

Preparation time: 45 minutes. Cooking equipment: saucepan.

Riata

Serves: 4

¼ cucumber
pinch of salt
1 medium tomato
1 small onion
200 g (7 oz) low-fat natural yoghurt
pepper
¼ tsp minced garlic
3-4 drops tabasco sauce

Method:

1. Peel and chop the cucumber. Sprinkle with salt. Place in sieve over bowl and allow to drain for 30 minutes.
2. Chop tomato and place in the second bowl.
3. Slice onion very finely.
4. Mix tomato, onion and cucumber.
5. Mix yoghurt, pepper, garlic and tabasco or chilli sauce.
6. Pour yoghurt mixture over vegetables, mix well, and refrigerate for an hour.

Nutrition data per serve: 174 kJ (42 cal), CHO 6 g, Protein 3 g, Fat 1 g.

Preparation time: 2 hours.

Crunchy Rice Salad

Serves: 4

2 cups cooked brown rice
½ green capsicum (bell pepper), chopped
½ red capsicum (bell pepper), chopped
4 spring onions (shallots), sliced
4 radishes, finely sliced
1 stick celery, finely sliced
¼ cup unsalted, roasted peanuts
½ cup canned water chestnuts, drained and sliced
½ cup green beans, lightly cooked
1 tbsp soy sauce
1 tsp sugar
2 tbsp chopped parsley
½ cup bean sprouts
pinch of salt, optional
garnish:
   spring onions (shallots), chopped radish slices

Method:

1. Combine all ingredients.
2. Chill.
3. Serve garnished with chopped spring onions (shallots) and radish slices.

Nutrition data per serve: 901 kJ (215 cal), CHO 35 g, Protein 7 g, Fat 5 g.
Preparation time: 30 minutes.

Tossed Salad

Serves: 4

¼ cup Italian Dressing (recipe, page 160) or commercial no-oil dressing

Use your imagination in creating tossed salads. For instance, consider blanched green beans, zucchini, broccoli florets, and cauliflower. You can combine alfalfa sprouts, mushrooms, snowpeas, sugar peas, carrot and celery with the more traditional ingredients such as various kinds of lettuce, capsicum (bell pepper), cucumber and tomatoes. Avocado adds a certain richness.

Sauces, Dressings and Marinades

SAUCES

White Sauce

Makes: 2 cups

2 cups skim milk
1 onion, cut in half
1 small carrot, roughly chopped
1 stalk celery, roughly chopped
6 peppercorns
2 tbsp cornflour (cornstarch)

Method:

1. Pour milk into saucepan. Add chopped vegetables and peppercorns.
2. Bring mixture to boil. Immediately reduce heat and simmer for 15 minutes.
3. Strain milk into a bowl. Discard vegetables and peppercorns.
4. In a separate bowl, mix cornflour (cornstarch) with 2 or 3 tbsp of the warm milk. Stir to make a smooth paste.
5. Gradually add remaining milk to the paste, stirring all the time.
6. Return sauce to the saucepan. Bring to boil, stirring constantly. Reduce heat and simmer gently for 2 minutes, stirring until sauce thickens.
7. Use as required in recipes.

Nutrition data per total quantity: 1036 kJ (247 cal), CHO 40 g, Protein 20 g, Fat 1 g.
Preparation time: 20 minutes. Cooking equipment: medium saucepan.

Cherry Sauce

Makes: 2 cups

2 cups fresh ripe cherries, pitted
½ cup Chicken Stock (recipe, page 71) (or ½ cup water and 1 stock cube)
1 tsp Worcestershire sauce
1 tbsp brandy

Method:

1. Place 1 cup of cherries into a saucepan or in a microwave bowl with stock and Worcestershire sauce.
2. Boil for 8 minutes until cherries are soft, or microwave on 'high' for 4 minutes. Purée and return to saucepan or bowl.
3. Add remaining cup of cherries and brandy. Simmer for 2 minutes or microwave on 'high' for 2 minutes, and serve.

Nutrition data per total quantity: 804 kJ (192 cal), CHO 48 g, Protein 2 g, Fat 0 g.
Preparation time: 15 minutes. Cooking equipment: saucepan.

Cheese Sauce

Makes: 2 cups

250 g (8 oz) cottage or ricotta cheese
½ cup grated low-fat block cheese
½ cup skim milk
1 tbsp cornflour (cornstarch)
1 tbsp skim milk, extra

This versatile and popular sauce works well with any number of savoury dishes. It is especially delicious with fish, vegetables or pasta. If you'd like a little more 'bite' to the sauce, add ½ tsp prepared English mustard and a pinch of cayenne pepper.

Method:

1. Using a food processor or electric blender, blend ricotta or cottage cheese and skim milk until smooth. Add the grated cheese.
2. In saucepan, gently warm the cheese mixture, stirring constantly, until the grated cheese melts.
3. In a cup, blend the cornflour (cornstarch) with the extra tablespoon of milk to make a smooth paste. Add to saucepan and stir into sauce.
4. Stirring constantly, bring sauce to the boil. Immediately reduce heat and simmer gently for 2 minutes, stirring constantly.

Nutrition data per total quantity: 2084 kJ (498 cal), CHO 21 g, Protein 66 g, Fat 18 g.
Preparation time: 10 minutes. Cooking equipment: medium saucepan, food processor or blender.

Saté (Peanut) Sauce

Makes: 2 cups

1 tbsp water
1 small onion, grated
1 clove garlic, crushed
½–1 tsp ground chilli
¾ cup crunchy peanut butter (preferably low-salt)
1 tbsp soy sauce
1 tbsp lemon juice
1¼ cups water

Method:

1. In a frying pan, bring water to the boil. Add onion and garlic and cook gently until soft.
2. Add chilli, stir in and cook for 1 minute over medium heat.
3. Add peanut butter and stir well. Add soy sauce, lemon juice and water and mix well. Bring mixture to boil, stirring constantly. Reduce heat and simmer gently for 1 minute.

Nutrition data per total quantity: 1548 kJ (370 cal), CHO 9 g, Protein 14 g, Fat 32 g.
Preparation time: 20 minutes. Cooking equipment: frying pan.

Fresh Vegetable Sauce

Makes: 4 cups

1 apple, peeled and grated
1 medium zucchini, grated
¼ medium green capsicum (bell pepper), finely chopped
1 small onion, finely chopped
2 medium tomatoes, finely chopped
3 medium mushrooms, finely chopped
1 medium carrot, grated
1 clove garlic, crushed
1 tbsp finely chopped parsley
½ tsp finely chopped fresh sage or ¼ tsp dried
½ tsp finely chopped fresh marjoram or ¼ tsp dried
ground black pepper
2 tbsp tomato paste
½ cup water

Method:

Place all ingredients in saucepan, bring to the boil and simmer for 20 minutes. Alternatively, place the ingredients in a microwave-proof bowl, and microwave on 'high' for 10 minutes.

Nutrition data per total quantity: 927 kJ (221 cal), CHO 40 g, Protein 14 g, Fat 1 g.

Preparation time: 30 minutes. Cooking equipment: medium saucepan.

Tomato and Basil Sauce

Serves: 4

2 tsp olive oil
1 medium onion, finely chopped
1 clove garlic, crushed
500 g (1 lb) ripe tomatoes, peeled, seeded and chopped
1 tbsp chopped fresh basil
½ tsp chopped fresh oregano
ground black pepper

Method:

1. Heat oil in saucepan, add onion and sauté until translucent.
2. Add garlic and cook for a further 2 minutes.
3. Add tomatoes, herbs and pepper and boil for 8-10 minutes.

Microwave method: Cooking time: 6-8 minutes

Sauté onion until soft (approximately 30 seconds). Add garlic and cook on 'high' for a further 1 minute. Add the tomatoes, herbs and pepper, and cook on 'high' for 4-6 minutes.

Nutrition data per total quantity: 793 kJ (190 cal), CHO 19 g, Protein 6 g, Fat 10 g.

Preparation time: 20 minutes. Cooking equipment: medium saucepan.

Black Bean Sauce

Makes: ½ cup

3 tbsp dried black beans
1 clove garlic, crushed
½ tsp finely chopped or minced fresh ginger (optional)
1 tbsp brandy or dry sherry
¼ cup water
2 tsp soy sauce

Delicious with finely sliced sautéed steak, chicken fillets or fish.

Method:

1. Wash beans thoroughly, drain and mash with garlic, ginger and brandy or sherry.
2. Place in saucepan with water and soy sauce.
3. Bring to the boil, reduce heat and simmer for 2 minutes.

Nutrition data per total quantity: 767 kJ (183 cal), CHO 16 g, Protein 15 g, Fat 8 g.

Preparation time: 7 minutes. Cooking equipment: small saucepan.

Ratatouille Sauce

Serves: 4

1 small green capsicum (bell pepper), diced
1 small eggplant (aubergine) peeled, diced
2 small zucchini, diced
2 medium tomatoes, diced, or 16 cherry tomatoes
6 medium mushrooms, diced
1 large onion, peeled and diced
1 clove garlic, crushed
½ tsp dried oregano
black pepper to taste
3 tbsp water

Ratatouille can be served as a hot vegetable or chilled as a salad. It is also ideal used to surround chicken, veal or fish fillets during cooking.

Method:

Combine all ingredients and cook over low heat for 30 minutes, or microwave on 'medium' for 15 minutes.

Nutrition data per total quantity: 184 kJ (44 cal), CHO 7 g, Protein 4 g, Fat 1 g.

Preparation time: 45 minutes. Cooking equipment: saucepan.

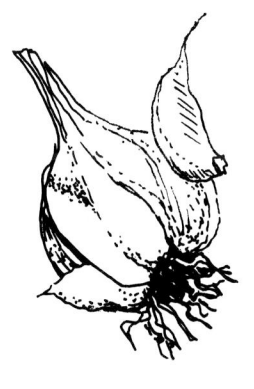

Cucumber and Yoghurt Sauce

Makes: 1 cup

½ cucumber, peeled
200 g (7 oz) low-fat natural yoghurt
1 tsp finely chopped or minced fresh ginger
½ tsp minced garlic
1 tbsp lemon juice
¼ tsp freshly ground black pepper
¼ tsp mild paprika
1 tbsp chopped parsley
4 cardamom pods, crushed

Use this sauce straightaway because it will not keep.

Method:

1. Grate cucumber, drain well and discard liquid.
2. Combine all the ingredients in a bowl and chill well before serving.

Nutrition data per total quantity: 514 kJ (123 cal), CHO 16 g, Protein 11 g, Fat 2 g.

Preparation time: 15 minutes.

Strawberry and Peppercorn Sauce

Makes: 2 cups

½ cup dry white wine
½ punnet strawberries, washed, hulled and puréed
1 tsp lemon juice
1 tsp brandy
2 tsp green or pink peppercorns
½ cup canned evaporated skim milk, chilled

Unusual but wonderful with grilled or sautéed chicken fillets, fish, lobster or crab.

Method:

1. Bring wine to the boil and reduce to half by simmering.
2. Add strawberry purée, lemon juice, brandy and peppercorns.
3. Bring back to the boil, simmer 1 minute and set it aside to cool.
4. Whip milk until it is thick. Gradually add the strawberry mixture to it, whipping constantly.
5. Gently reheat the mixture, but do not allow it to boil. Serve immediately.

Nutrition data per total quantity: 200 kJ (48 cal), CHO 7 g, Protein 5 g, Fat trace.

Preparation time: 15 minutes. Cooking equipment: medium saucepan.

Sweet and Sour Sauce

This is a wonderfully versatile sauce that is just as good served with boiled brown rice or noodles, as it is served with grilled fish, pork or vegetables.

Serves: 4

1 large onion
8 spring onions (shallots)
2 medium carrots
1 small red capsicum (bell pepper), deseeded
125 g (4 oz) mushrooms
2 sticks celery
1 medium cucumber
2 tsp oil
1 clove garlic, crushed
1 tsp grated or minced fresh ginger
2 tbsp tomato paste
¼ cup white vinegar
1 cup water
1 stock cube
1½ tbsp cornflour (cornstarch)
3 tbsp soy sauce
1 tbsp dry sherry
400 g (14 oz) can of unsweetened canned pineapple pieces and juice

Method:

1. Slice onion, spring onions (shallots), capsicum (bell pepper), mushrooms, and celery thinly (about matchstick size).
2. Cut cucumbers into quarters, lengthwise, remove seeds and cut into small pieces of about 1½ cm (½ in).
3. Heat oil in a large wok or frying pan over high heat. Add garlic and ginger. Stir-fry for 30 seconds, and then add all the other vegetables. Keep heat high and stir-fry for 2-3 minutes until the vegetables are cooked, but still crisp and bright coloured.
4. In a bowl, blend tomato paste, vinegar, water, stock cube, cornflour (cornstarch), soy sauce and sherry.
5. Drain pineapple pieces, and add the juice to the tomato paste mixture. Keep pineapple aside. Add sauce mixture to the vegetables, and stir until sauce boils and thickens.
6. Add pineapple to the vegetables, and cook for another 3-5 minutes until the pineapple is heated through.

To serve: As an accompaniment: serve hot or cold with grilled fish (method, page 87), or pork and Vegetables en Brochette (recipe, page 141). As a light meal: serve the sauce with boiled brown rice or noodles.

Nutrition data per total quantity: 2163 kJ (517 cal), CHO 87 g, Protein 17 g, Fat 11 g.

Preparation time: 30 minutes. Cooking equipment: wok or frying pan.

Green Champagne Sauce

Makes: 1 cup

3 kiwifruit, peeled and puréed
½ cup halved sultana grapes
½ cup champagne

Simple, sophisticated and superb, especially with fish.

Method:

1. Place kiwifruit in saucepan. Add grapes and champagne.
2. Heat gently, but do not boil. Serve immediately.

Nutrition data per total quantity: 1210 kJ (289 cal), CHO 46 g, Protein 5 g, Fat 1 g.

Preparation time: 10 minutes. Equipment: small-medium saucepan.

DRESSINGS

Italian Dressing

Makes: ½ cup

1/3 cup vinegar
1 tbsp lemon juice
1 tbsp chopped parsley
2 tsp chopped chives
1 clove garlic, crushed
½ tsp dry mustard
ground black pepper

Method:

Combine ingredients in a screw top jar, shake well and refrigerate.

To store: cover and refrigerate for up to one week.

Nutrition data per total quantity: negligible
Preparation time: 5 minutes.

Creamy Yoghurt Dressing

Makes: ½ cup

1/3 cup low-fat natural yoghurt
2 tbsp lemon juice or raspberry vinegar
½ tsp dry mustard
ground black pepper

Method:

Mix all ingredients until smooth. Cover and refrigerate.

To store: cover and refrigerate for up to three days.

Nutrition data per total quantity: 189 kJ (45cal), CHO 6 g, Protein 4 g, Fat 1 g.
Preparation time: 5 minutes.

Orange and Soy Dressing

Makes: ¼ cup

¼ cup unsweetened orange juice
2 tsp soy sauce
1 clove garlic, crushed
1 tsp oil (optional)

Method:

1. Combine all ingredients in a screw top jar.
2. Chill and shake well before use.

To store: cover and refrigerate for up to two days.

Nutrition data per total quantity: 269kJ (64 cal), CHO 4 g, Protein trace, Fat 5 g.
Preparation time: 5 minutes.

Foreground: Corn Chowder, centre left, Apple Layer Cake and centre right Meatloaf with Spicy Barbecue Sauce.

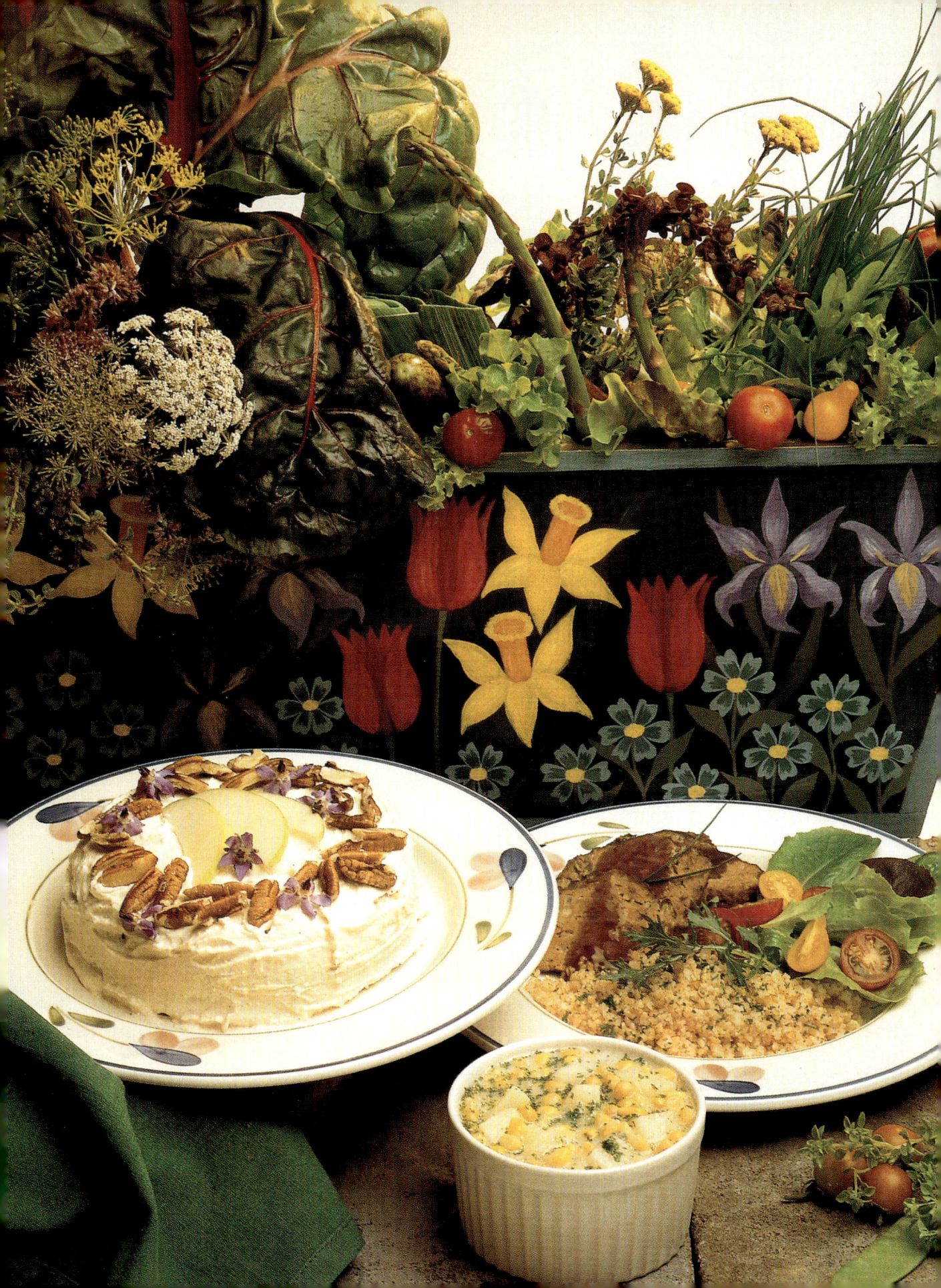

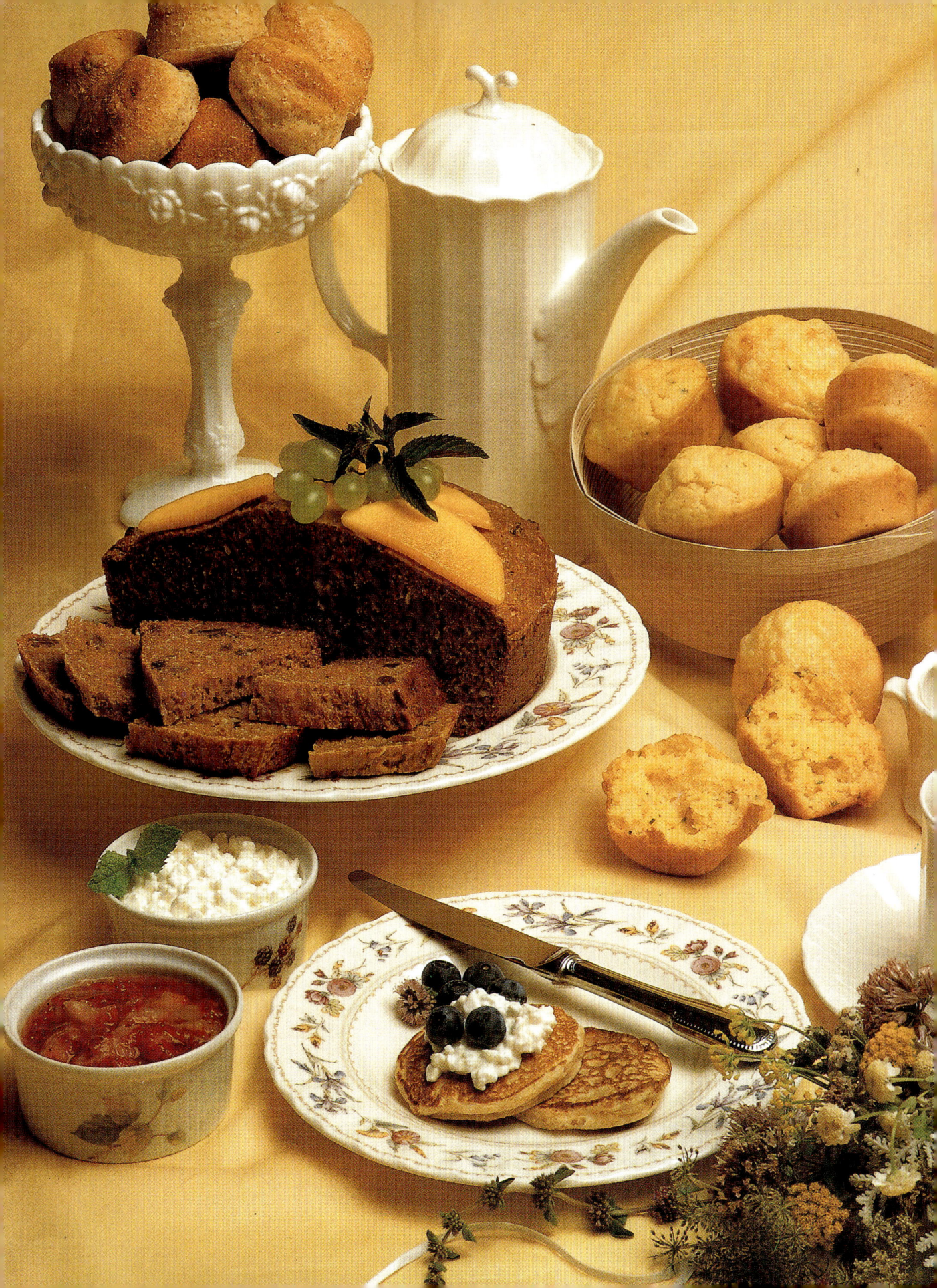

Herbed Tomato Dressing

Makes: 1 cup

½ cup unsweetened tomato juice
4 tbsp tomato paste
2 tbsp low-fat natural yoghurt
4 drops tabasco sauce
1 clove garlic, crushed
1 tbsp chopped parsley
½ tsp chopped fresh mixed herbs or ¼ tsp mixed dried herbs

Use herbs such as marjoram, basil or thyme.

Method:

1. Combine tomato juice with tomato paste and add to yoghurt.
2. Add other ingredients and mix well.
3. Chill and use same day.

Nutrition data per total quantity: 411 kJ (98 cal), CHO 16 g, Protein 8 g, Fat trace.

Preparation time: 8 minutes.

Creamy Orange Dressing

Makes: ¾ cup

¼ cup unsweetened orange juice
2 tsp grated orange rind
1 tbsp finely chopped parsley
2 tsp finely chopped chives
½ cup low-fat natural yoghurt

Method:

Combine all ingredients and chill.

To vary: for creamy lemon dressing, prepare as above but omit orange juice and rind, replacing them with 2 tbsp lemon juice.

To store: cover and refrigerate for up to two days.

Nutrition data per total quantity: 421 kJ (101 cal), CHO 14 g, Protein 8 g, Fat 2 g.

Preparation time: 5 minutes.

Curry Dressing

Makes: ½ cup

½ cup low-fat natural yoghurt
2 tsp hot Curry Powder or Paste (recipe, page 164)
2 tbsp chopped parsley
¼ tsp minced garlic (optional)

Method:

1. Mix all ingredients and adjust flavourings to taste.
2. Chill and use same day.

Nutrition data per total quantity: 337 kJ (80 cal), CHO 9 g, Protein 8 g, Fat 2 g.

Preparation time: 5 minutes.

Foreground: Pikelets and Fresh Strawberry Conserve, centre, Carrot Cake with a basket of Herby Corn Muffins, and Wholemeal Scones at top.

QUICK AND EASY MARINADES

Try these marinades with lean beef steaks, lamb cutlets, pork schnitzel or as a marinade for meat to place on skewers. Excellent for barbecue or grill. These quantities are for 500 g (1 lb) of meat and will serve four.

Red Wine Zap: Combine ½ cup dry red wine, 1 tbsp tomato paste, 1 tbsp Worcestershire (or soy or teriyaki) sauce, 2 tbsp finely chopped parsley, 1 clove crushed garlic, ground black pepper to taste and ¼ tsp finely chopped oregano or basil (optional).

To rev it up — add ¼ cup sweet chilli sauce, ¼ cup Worcestershire sauce, or 1-2 cloves crushed garlic. Stir ingredients, and use to brush meat as it grills.

Singapore Sizzler: Combine 1 tbsp Worcestershire sauce, 1 tbsp soy or teriyaki sauce, 2 tbsp lemon juice, ¼ tsp mustard powder, ¼ tsp ground coriander and ¼ tsp finely chopped green ginger. Stir the ingredients and use to brush meat as it grills.

Spicy Lamb: Particularly good for lamb is a combination of ½ cup tomato paste, 2 tsp Worcestershire sauce, 2 tsp chopped fresh or ½ tsp dried rosemary, dash of tabasco sauce and 4 chopped spring onions (shallots). Stir the ingredients and use to brush meat as it grills.

PICKLES AND SEASONINGS

Tomato Relish

Makes: 8 cups

3 large onions
2½ kg (5½ lb) chopped, ripe tomatoes
5 granny smith apples, cored and chopped (skins left on)
3 cups vinegar
500 g (1 lb) sultanas
3 gloves of garlic, crushed
1 cup fresh orange juice
1 tsp mixed spice
1 tsp whole cloves
1 tsp chilli powder

Method:

1. Place all the ingredients in a large saucepan and bring them to the boil. Turn the heat to low and simmer for 1 hour, stirring frequently. Remove from heat.
2. Pour hot water into clean jars to warm them. Pour water away.
3. Fill jars with hot chutney. Allow them to cool, then seal the jars and store.

To store: keep in sealed jars. Once opened, store in refrigerator.

Nutrition data per total quantity: 8820 kJ (2107 cal), CHO 503 g, Protein 42 g, Fat 1 g.

Preparation time: 1½ hours. Cooking equipment: large saucepan.

Fresh Mango Pickle

Makes: ¾-1 cup

1 ripe medium-large mango
2 tsp lemon juice
½ tsp finely chopped or minced fresh ginger
1 tbsp sultanas

Method:

1. Peel mango. Slice flesh from stone and cut into small pieces. Place in a mixing bowl.
2. Add lemon juice, ginger, and sultanas.
3. Spoon into glass or plastic container, cover and refrigerate.

To store: keep in glass or plastic container and refrigerate for up to two days.

Nutrition data per total quantity: 425 kJ (102 cal), CHO 24 g, Protein 2 g, Fat trace.
Preparation time: 15 mins.

Plum Sauce

Makes: 8 cups

2 onions, chopped
1 cup water
1 kg (2 lb) fresh plums, stoned
1 cup fresh orange juice
2 tsp grated or minced fresh ginger
½ tsp whole cloves
¼ tsp peppercorns
pinch of thyme
pinch of oregano
1 bay leaf

Method:

1. Lightly sauté onions in 2-3 tablespoons of the water, for 2 minutes.
2. Add the rest of the ingredients and cook over low heat, stirring regularly.
3. Simmer, with the lid off for at least 1 hour until the mixture thickens.
4. Pour into clean warmed jars, allow to cool and then seal.

To store: keep in sealed jars in refrigerator.

Nutrition data per total quantity: 2238 kJ (545 cal), CHO 124 g, Protein 12 g, Fat 1 g.
Preparation time: 1½ hours. Cooking equipment: large saucepan.

Curry Paste

Makes: ¾ *cup*

1 tbsp freshly minced or grated ginger
2 tbsp ground coriander
1 tbsp ground cinnamon
2 tsp chilli powder
1 tbsp powdered turmeric
1 tsp minced garlic
1 tbsp lemon juice
2 tbsp vinegar
2 tbsp oil
1 tbsp seeded mustard

You can vary the quantities and ingredients according to taste.

Method:

1. Combine ingredients in saucepan and mix to make a smooth paste.
2. Stirring constantly, cook over low heat for 3-4 minutes until slightly thickened.
3. Spoon mixture into a warmed glass jar, seal and store in refrigerator.

To store: keep in airtight container in refrigerator for up to one month.

Nutrition data per total quantity: negligible

Preparation time: 6 minutes. Cooking equipment: saucepan.

Curry Powder

Makes: ¾ *cup*

½ tsp cayenne pepper
2 tbsp ground coriander
1 tbsp ground cumin
1 tbsp coarsely ground black pepper
2 tbsp ground ginger
1 tbsp ground cinnamon
½ tsp ground cloves
¼ tsp ground nutmeg
2 tsp chilli powder
2 tbsp powdered turmeric

You can vary the ingredients and quantities according to taste. Curry Powder can be stored for a long time, but gradually loses its flavour.

Method:

1. Mix ingredients well.
2. Refrigerate in airtight container.

Nutrition data per total quantity: negligible.

Preparation time: 15 minutes.

SWEET SAUCES

Creamy Whipped Topping

Makes: 2 cups

½ cup skim milk powder
1 cup iced water
½ tsp vanilla

Mixture will lose its thickness after 2-3 hours, just re-whip it.

Method:

1. Combine all ingredients in a bowl.
2. With electric beater, hand beater or whisk, beat mixture until thick and creamy. Chill.

Nutrition data per total quantity: 680 kJ (163 cal), CHO 24 g, Protein 16 g, Fat 1 g.
Preparation time: 10 minutes.

Blueberry Sauce

Serves: 4

1 cup blueberries, fresh or frozen
½ cup orange juice
½ tsp cinnamon
1 tbsp brown sugar
2 tsp cornflour (cornstarch)
1 tbsp water

Method:

1. Place berries, juice, cinammon, and sugar into a saucepan. Bring to the boil, then remove from heat.
2. Combine cornflour (cornstarch) and water, making sure there are no lumps.
3. Stir into the berries, then reheat until the mixture thickens.
4. Spoon hot sauce over pancakes.

Nutrition data per serve: 217 kJ (52 cal), CHO 13 g, Protein 0.4 g, Fat trace.
Peparation time: 15 minutes. Cooking equipment: saucepan.

Custard Sauce

Serves: 4

3 level tbsp custard powder
500 ml (18 fl oz) skim milk
1 tsp vanilla
2 tsp sugar, Equal™ or other artificial sweetener

You can serve this sauce hot or cold.

Method:

1. Blend custard powder and a small quantity of the milk to make a smooth paste.
2. Place remaining milk in saucepan and bring to boil.
3. Gradually stir in custard paste. Continue stirring until mixture thickens.
4. Simmer for 1 minute, stirring constantly.
5. Add vanilla and sugar, Equal™ or other artificial sweetener.

Nutrition data per serve: 298 kJ (71 cal), CHO 13 g, Protein 5 g, Fat trace.
Preparation time: 15 minutes. Cooking equipment: saucepan.

Orange Custard Sauce

Follow the recipe for custard sauce and add 1 tsp of finely grated orange rind to milk before heating.

Brandy Sauce

Serves: 4

1 quantity of Custard Sauce (recipe above)
1 egg, separated
2 tbsp brandy

Method:

1. Beat egg yolk and add to custard sauce.
3. Whip egg white until peaks form.
4. Fold egg white through custard and add brandy.
5. Serve immediately.

Nutrition data per serve: 462 kJ (110 cal), CHO 13 g, Protein 6 g, Fat 1 g.
Preparation time: 20 minutes. Cooking equipment: saucepan.

Desserts

Apple Layer Cake

Serves: 10-12

Biscuits:
cup wholemeal
  self-raising flour
125 g (4 oz) low-fat
  cream cheese
1 egg
1 tsp vanilla essence
2 tsp brown sugar

Filling:
2½ cups cold, stewed
  apple, flavoured with
  lemon rind, cinnamon
  and cloves to taste

Topping:
125 g (4 oz) low-fat
  cream cheese
2 tsp sugar
rind ½ lemon, finely
  grated
125 g (4 oz) ricotta
  cheese
¼ tsp ground cinnamon

Decoration:
50 g (2 oz) chopped
  pecans

Refrigerate this glorious cake for a day before you serve it so that it is easy to cut and the filling has developed its full flavour.

Method:

Biscuits:
1. Sift flour into bowl. Return bran to sifted flour.
2. Soften cheese, and beat with a spoon until smooth. Add egg and vanilla and beat again. Add sugar and mix well.
3. Gradually blend flour into cheese mixture until a soft dough is formed.
4. Turn out onto a floured board and knead into a ball.
5. Divide into three. Shape and roll into rounds approximately 25 cm (10 in) in diameter, making them as equal as possible.
6. Lift onto very lightly greased baking trays.
7. Bake for 12 minutes until cooked through and light brown.
8. Remove and cool on cake racks

Filling:
9. Add lemon rind, cinnamon and cloves (to taste) to cold, stewed apple. Mixture should be fairly firm.

Topping:
10. Soften low-fat cream cheese until smooth. Add sugar, lemon rind, ricotta and cinnamon and mix well.

Assembly:
13. Place one biscuit round on serving plate. Cover with half the apple. Cover with the second round, spread with the remainder of the apple, then place third round on top.
14. Spread topping mixture on top and sides of cake.
15. Sprinkle with pecans, cover with plastic film and refrigerate for at least 24 hours.
16. Cut into wedges to serve.

Nutrition data per serve (if 10 serves): 763 kJ (182 cal), CHO 17 g, Protein 6 g, Fat 10 g.
Preparation time: biscuits 30 minutes, assembly 30 minutes, begin preparation 24 hours before serving. Cooking equipment: 2 baking trays. Oven temperature: 180°C (350°F).

Fruit Strudel

Apple Strudel
Serves: 4

6 sheets filo pastry
2 tbsp skim milk
4 apples, peeled and sliced very finely
4 tbsp sultanas
2 tbsp chopped pecan nuts
1 tsp cinnamon
¼ tsp ground cloves
1 tbsp brown sugar

All the pleasure of the traditional strudel, but with a fraction of the fat.

Method:

1. Spread out 2 sheets of pastry on a kitchen bench. Brush lightly with milk.
2. Place another 2 layers of pastry on top. Again brush with milk.
3. Repeat for remaining two sheets of pastry.
4. Sprinkle remaining ingredients over the pastry.
5. Spray a baking tray with non-stick baking spray. Carefully roll up the pastry. Place on the baking tray, loose edge down.
6. Brush the strudel well with milk. Bake for 25-30 minutes.

Serve warm, cut in thick slices. You may serve this with Creamy Whipped Topping (recipe, page 165).

Nutrition data per serve: 800 kJ (191 cal), CHO 36 g, Protein 5 g, Fat 5 g.
Preparation time: 45 minutes. Cooking equipment: baking tray. Oven temperature: 200°C (400°F).

Banana Strudel

The basic method is exactly the same as for Apple Strudel (see above); only the filling is different. For this delectable filling combine:
4 ripe bananas (sliced), 4 tbsp sultanas, 1 tsp cinnamon, 4 tbsp shredded coconut, 2 tbsp unsweetened orange juice, 2 tbsp chopped pecan nuts or walnuts, 4 tbsp brown rum and 1 tsp brown sugar.

Nutrition data per serve: 1102 kJ (263 cal), CHO 43 g, Protein 7 g, Fat 9 g.

Apricot Strudel

The basic method is exactly the same as for Apple Strudel (see above); only the filling is different. Here you combine:
500 g (1 lb) apricots (stoned and sliced) or 1 can (425 g/15 oz) of unsweetened apricot pieces, 4 tbsp sultanas, 2 tbsp slivered almonds, 1 tsp cinnamon and 1 tbsp brown sugar.

Nutrition data per serve: 580 kJ (138 cal), CHO 22 g, Protein 5 g, Fat 5 g.

Ricotta Raisin Flan

Serves: 6-8

2 tbsp margarine
125 g (4 oz) shredded wheatmeal biscuits, crushed
500 g (1 lb) ricotta cheese
4 tbsp apple concentrate
1 cup raisins, chopped
rind of 1 lemon, grated
½ tsp ground cinnamon
¼ tsp ground nutmeg
1 egg
½ cup low-fat milk
garnish: ground cinnamon

Method:

1. Melt margarine, then pour into biscuit crumbs and mix.
2. Spread over base and up sides of pie dish. Press well to make an even, firm crust.
3. Bake 10 minutes. Cool.
4. Mix ricotta, apple concentrate, raisins, lemon rind and spices.
5. Beat egg and combine with milk. Mix it with other ingredients. Blend well.
6. Pour into pie dish. Bake for 30-45 minutes until set and lightly browned.
7. Sprinkle with a little cinnamon and serve.

To store: cover and refrigerate for up to two days.

Nutrition data per serve: 1562 kJ (373 cal), CHO 43 g, Protein 13 g, Fat 17 g.

Preparation time: 1 hour 50 minutes. Cooking equipment: small saucepan, pie dish. Oven temperature: 180°C (350°F).

Lemon Delicious

Serves: 4

3 eggs
5 tbsp fresh lemon juice
rind of 1 lemon, freshly grated
1 tbsp melted butter
3 tbsp wholemeal plain flour
1½ cups low-fat milk
1 tbsp sugar or Sweetaddin™

Method:

1. Separate eggs. Beat egg whites until stiff peaks form.
2. Beat yolks with the remaining ingredients until smooth.
3. Gradually fold the egg whites into mixture.
4. Spoon evenly into four dishes.
5. Place in a larger baking dish. Carefully pour water into the larger baking dish until it reaches two-thirds up the outside of the individual baking dishes.
6. Bake for approximately 20 minutes or until set and lightly browned.
7. Cool slightly in the water-filled dish to prevent shrinking.

To store: cover and refrigerate for 1 day only.

Nutrition data per serve: 886 kJ (212 cal), CHO 12 g, Protein 9 g, Fat 14 g.

Preparation time: 1 hour. Cooking equipment: individual baking dishes, large baking dish for water bath. Oven temperature: 160°C (325°F).

Spiced Oranges

Serves: 4

1 cup red wine, such as claret or burgundy
½ cup unsweetened orange juice
¼ tsp ground cinnamon or 1 cinnamon stick
3 oranges
Equal™ or other artificial sweetener to taste

The ideal dessert after a long hot summer's day.

Method:

1. Place wine, orange juice and cinnamon in a saucepan and bring to the boil.
2. Boil hard for 2 minutes, then remove from heat, or microwave on 'high' for 2-3 minutes.
3. Peel and thinly slice oranges, removing all pith and seeds, and arrange in a glass serving bowl.
4. Pour wine mixture over oranges, discarding cinnamon stick if used.
5. Chill well and sweeten before serving.

To store: cover and refrigerate for up to four days.

Nutrition data per serve: 219 kJ (52 cal), CHO 11 g, Protein 1 g, Fat trace.
Preparation time: 15 minutes. Cooking equipment: saucepan.

Creamy Rice

Serves: 4

1 cup uncooked basmati rice
1½ cups water
2½ cups skim or low-fat milk
½ cup sultanas
½ tsp ground nutmeg
1 tsp vanilla essence
2 sachets of Equal™ or artificial sweetener equivalent to 4 tsp of sugar

Method:

1. Wash rice and place in saucepan, cover with the water, and simmer over very low heat until water is absorbed.
2. Add 1 cup milk. Simmer again until absorbed.
3. Add the remaining 1½ cups milk and cook again until the milk is absorbed.
4. Stir in sultanas, nutmeg, vanilla and sweetener (to taste).
5. Serve warm with sliced stewed or fresh fruit.

To store: cover and refrigerate for up to three days.

Nutrition data per serve: 1185 kJ (283 cal), CHO 58 g, Protein 10 g, Fat 1 g.
Preparation time: 1 hour. Cooking equipment: saucepan.

Sweet Potato and Pecan Pie

Serves: 8

15 shredded wheatmeal biscuits, crushed
3 tbsp margarine, melted
2 cups mashed cooked sweet potato (kumara)
4 tbsp lemon juice
1 tsp cinnamon
¼ tsp mixed spice
¼ tsp ground ginger
3 tbsp brown sugar
pinch salt
1 cup low-fat milk
125 g (4 oz) pecan kernels
2 eggs, separated

Method:

1. Line a pie or flan dish with aluminium foil.
2. Mix crushed biscuits with margarine and spoon into dish. Spread over base and up the sides, pressing with the back of a spoon.
3. Bake for 10-15 minutes, then remove and cool.
4. Spoon sweet potato into a mixing bowl. Add lemon juice, cinnamon, mixed spice, ginger, sugar, and salt and stir well to combine.
5. Stir in milk, pecan kernels, and egg yolks.
6. Beat egg whites until soft peaks form, then fold into sweet potato mixture.
7. Spoon into crumb crust and bake for 45-60 minutes, or until set and lightly browned. Serve warm or cold.

Nutrition data per portion: 1439 kJ (344 cal), CHO 31 g, Protein 7 g, Fat 22 g.

Preparation time: 1½ hours. Cooking equipment: saucepan, pie dish. Oven temperature: 180°C (350°F).

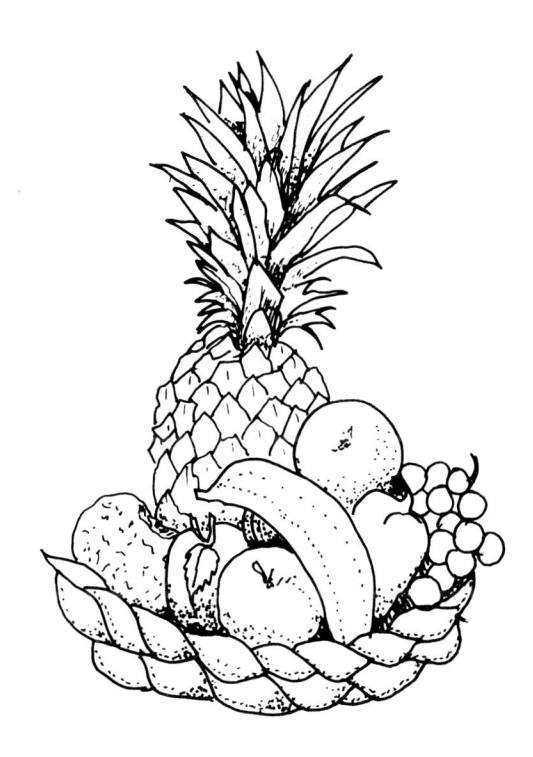

Fruit Crumble

Serves: 4

3 large cooking apples, peeled cored and sliced
2 tbsp water
½ tsp ground cinnamon or 3 cloves
Topping:
1⅓ cups Meg's Muesli (recipe, page 58)
or
½ cup rolled oats
2 tbsp desiccated coconut
2 tbsp mixed dried fruit
2 tsp chopped nuts
¼ cup wheatflakes
¼ cup all-bran

You can replace the apples in this recipe with peaches, apricots or plums or with two apples and half a cup of cooked rhubarb. If you have a favourite combination, you can use it in this recipe, too.

Method:

1. Place apple into a saucepan, add water and cinnamon or cloves.
2. Gently simmer for approximately 10 minutes until apple is tender, or microwave, covered, on 'high' for 6 minutes.
3. Lightly grease a small casserole and spoon in apple, removing cloves if used.
4. Mix topping ingredients and sprinkle thickly over apple.
5. Bake for 30 minutes or until topping becomes golden.
6. Serve hot or cold.

To store: cover and refrigerate for up to 4 days.

Nutrition data per serve: 1025 kJ (245 cal), CHO 38 g, Protein 7 g, Fat 7 g.

Preparation time: 1 hour. Cooking equipment: saucepan, small casserole. Oven temperature: 180°C (350°F).

Summer Pudding

Serves: 4

14 slices wholemeal bread
6 cups mixed fresh berries (strawberries, raspberries, blueberries, loganberries)
4 tsp castor sugar
garnish: extra berries

Method:

1. Cut crusts off bread and discard them.
2. Cut 4 round bases and tops out of crustless bread. Set tops aside. Place a base in each individual soufflé dish. Use the remaining bread to line the sides of the dishes. Do this carefully, making sure that there are no gaps.
3. Wash and hull berries. Chop strawberries.
4. Place berries and sugar in saucepan, and heat gently until liquid runs from berries.
5. Fill soufflé dishes, packing fruit down firmly, and pour juice over.
6. Cover each with one of the reserved tops.

7. Place a weight on top and refrigerate overnight.
8. Remove and discard the tops.
9. Turn onto serving dishes. Garnish with extra berries.

Nutrition data per serve: 876 kJ (209 cal), CHO 42 g, Protein 7 g, Fat 1 g.

Preparation time: 20 minutes, plus overnight standing time. Cooking equipment: 4 individual soufflé dishes, saucepan.

Pumpkin Pie

Serves: 6

Pastry:

2 tbsp margarine

1 cup wholemeal flour

1 egg yolk

juice of ½ lemon plus cold water to make ⅓ cup

Filling:

2 cups firm pumpkin purée

¼ cup ricotta cheese

¼ cup low-fat natural yoghurt

½ cup skim or low-fat milk

2 eggs, separated

¼ tsp nutmeg

¼ tsp mixed spice

½ tsp cinnamon

juice and grated rind of 1 lemon

Equal™ or other artificial sweetener to taste

garnish: ground cinnamon

This is simply delicious.

Method:

Pastry:
1. Rub margarine into flour until mixture resembles fine breadcrumbs.
2. Mix egg yolk with juice and water.
3. Mix liquid into flour with a knife, to make a soft dough.
4. Turn out onto floured board. Knead lightly, leave for 15 mins.
5. Roll out on floured board, then cover base and sides of pie dish with pastry. Add a second strip around the top edge and pinch as a decorative edge. Prick pastry and place in oven, bake for approximately 1 hour until lightly browned. Remove and cool.

Filling:
6. Combine in a bowl pumpkin, ricotta, yoghurt, milk, and egg yolks. Beat well.
7. Add spices, lemon juice and rind, and sweetener. Check taste and adjust if necessary.
8. Beat egg whites until soft peaks form, fold into pumpkin mixture.
9. Pour into pastry shell and bake in a preheated oven until set (about 1 hour).
10. Sprinkle with a little cinnamon to serve.

To vary: fold ¼ cup chopped pecans into filling.

To store: cover and refrigerate for up to two days.

Nutrition data per serve: 851 kJ (203 cal), CHO 20 g, Protein 9 g, Fat 10 g.

Preparation time: 2 hours. Cooking equipment: pie dish. Oven temperature: 180°C (350°F).

Mixed Berry Salad with Lemon Cream

Serves: 4

Salad:
1 punnet or 250 g (8 oz) strawberries
1 punnet or 250 g (8 oz) blackberries
1 punnet or 250 g (8 oz) blueberries
¼ cup unsweetened apple juice
Lemon cream:
250 g (8 oz) ricotta cheese
100 g (3 oz) low-fat natural yoghurt
rind of 1 lemon, grated
2 tsp brown sugar

When berries are in season, celebrate with this salad dressed with smooth lemon cream.

Method:

1. Wash and hull berries, slice strawberries if large.
2. Place in bowl and pour apple juice over.
3. Chill in refrigerator.

Lemon cream:

4. Mix ricotta, yoghurt, lemon rind and sugar.
5. Chill.
6. Spoon lemon cream over fruit and serve.

To vary: replace blackberries with loganberries.

Nutrition data per serve: 419 kJ (100 cal), CHO 20 g, Protein 4 g, Fat 1 g.

Preparation time: 30 minutes.

Hot Jamaican Pineapple

Serves: 4

½ medium pineapple, cut lengthwise with top intact
3 bananas, peeled and chopped
4 tsp brown rum
2 tsp brown sugar
¼ cup shredded desiccated coconut

Method:

1. Cut pineapple out of skin, being careful not to pierce skin. Scoop out any remaining pulp and juice and retain.
2. Chop pineapple into chunks, discarding core. Add to pulp and juice in bowl. Add bananas. Add rum and brown sugar.
3. Spoon fruit and juices into shell and sprinkle with coconut.
4. Place in baking dish, and bake for 30-45 minutes until fruit is heated through and coconut is toasted.
5. Spoon into serving dishes.

Nutrition data per serve: 542 kJ (130 cal), CHO 25 g, Protein 2 g, Fat 2 g.

Preparation time: 1 hour. Cooking equipment: baking dish. Oven temperature: 180°C (350°F).

Ginger Pears

Serves: 4

4 medium pears, peeled and quartered
285 ml (10 fl oz) bottle low-joule (low-calorie) dry ginger ale
juice of 1 lemon
½ tsp minced fresh ginger
¼ cup orange juice concentrate
3-4 drops yellow food colouring (optional)
6 cloves
garnish: ground cinnamon

Method:

1. Place pears in saucepan. Add dry ginger ale, lemon juice, ginger, orange juice concentrate, food colouring and cloves.
2. Cover and simmer until pears are tender, turning and basting the pears so they cook and colour evenly. Alternatively microwave, covered, on 'high' for 4-6 minutes until tender.
3. Lift pears onto serving dish.
4. Simmer juice until slightly reduced.
5. Pour over pears. Sprinkle with cinnamon.
6. Serve hot or chilled.

To store: cover and refrigerate for up to four days.

Nutrition data per serve: 382 kJ (91 cal), CHO 22 g, Protein 1 g, Fat 0 g.

Preparation time: 1 hour. Cooking equipment: saucepan.

Fruity Baked Rice Pudding

Serves: 4

3½ cups skim milk
5 tbsp uncooked brown or white rice
1 tbsp sugar
4 tbsp sultanas or raisins
4 tbsp dried peaches or apricots
garnish: ground nutmeg or cinnamon

Method:

1. Combine milk, rice and sugar.
2. Place mixture in baking dish.
3. Cover and bake for 45 minutes.
4. Remove from oven, add dried fruit and stir.
5. Leave uncovered and return to oven. Cook for another 45-60 minutes until rice is cooked. A skin will form on top of rice.
6. Serve hot or cold, garnished with ground nutmeg or cinnamon.

To store: cover and refrigerate or up to three days.

Nutrition data per serve: 1191 kJ (284 cal), CHO 60 g, Protein 11 g, Fat trace.

Preparation time: 2 hours. Cooking equipment: baking dish with lid. Oven temperature: 180°C (350°F).

Old-Fashioned Dumplings

Serves: 4

3/4 cup skim or low-fat milk
1/4 tsp ground nutmeg
1/2 cup semolina
1 egg
1 tsp vanilla essence
1 tbsp mixed peel
1 tbsp currants
1 tbsp sultanas
small quantity of plain flour
1 cup Orange Custard Sauce (recipe, page 166) or 1 cup apple purée

Method:

1. Place milk and nutmeg in small saucepan and bring to boil.
2. Remove from heat and quickly stir in semolina.
3. Return to heat and stir for one minute.
4. Add egg, vanilla, peel, currants and sultanas and mix well.
5. Turn onto a lightly floured board and knead gently till smooth.
6. Break off small, even-sized pieces and roll into balls the size of large marbles. Toss each ball in flour.
7. Half fill a large saucepan with water and bring to boil.
8. Drop dumplings into boiling water and cook for approximately 5 minutes. (Note: the dumplings will rise to the top of the water as they cook.)
9. Drain and serve immediately with orange custard sauce or apple purée.

Nutrition data per serve: 584 kJ (140 cal), CHO 24 g, Protein 7 g, Fat 2 g.
Preparation time: 20 minutes plus preparation time for sauce. Cooking equipment: small saucepan, large saucepan.

Baked Apples with Orange and Strawberry Sauce

Serves: 4

4 granny smith apples
cinnamon
1 cup orange juice
1 punnet strawberries
liquid artificial sweetener to taste
2 tbsp slivered almonds or chopped pecans
orange slices

Method:

1. Peel and core apples. When peeling leave some peel on to create a horizontal striped effect.
2. Place in a small baking dish. Sprinkle cinnamon over, then orange juice.
3. Bake, covered, for 30-35 minutes, or microwave on 'high' for 6-8 minutes, until tender but still retaining their shape. Baste occasionally to prevent drying out.
4. While apples are cooking, wash and hull strawberries and purée them. Add sweetener to purée.
5. When apples are cooked, lift gently onto individual serving dishes.

6. Reduce cooking liquid by boiling if necessary, and pour into strawberry purée. Mix and pour over apples.
7. Decorate with slivered nuts and orange slices.
8. Serve warm or chilled.

To store: cover and refrigerate for up to two days.

Nutrition data per serve: 387 kJ (92 cal), CHO 18 g, Protein 2 g, Fat 1 g.
Preparation time: 1 hour. Cooking equipment: food processor, baking dish, small saucepan. Oven temperature: 180°C (350°F).

English Fruit Compote

Serves: 4

1 small apple, peeled, cored and cut into 8 wedges
1 cup unsweetened canned peaches in natural juice, made up of approximately ½ cup peaches and ½ cup liquid
1 small pear, peeled, cored and cut into 8 wedges
12 whole cherries
4 yellow plums, cut into half and stoned
2 cloves
pinch ground cinnamon

This is usually a chilled dessert, but you can serve it hot. Vary the fruit according to season and your preference. For instance, if fresh plums are not available, use canned, unsweetened apricot halves or peach slices which you add after the other fruit has been cooked.

Method:
1. Place ingredients in saucepan, with apple at the bottom and peaches on the top.
2. Bring to the boil and simmer gently for 10 minutes or until all fruit is tender.
3. Cool and place in refrigerator for at least 2 hours before serving in glass dishes.

To store: cover and refrigerate for up to three days.

Microwave method:

Place fruit in microwave dish, cover and cook on 'medium' for 5 minutes.

Nutrition data per serve: 283 kJ (68 cal), CHO 16 g, Protein 1 g, Fat 0 g.
Preparation time: 2 hours 20 minutes, including cooling time. Cooking equipment: medium saucepan.

Baked Custard

Serves: 4

2 eggs
liquid artificial sweetener to taste
1⅓ cups skim milk
1 tsp vanilla essence
sprinkling of ground nutmeg

This family favourite can be served hot or cold.

Method:

1. In bowl, lightly beat the eggs.
2. Gradually add the milk to the egg mixture, stirring constantly. Stir in the vanilla essence and sweetener. Check flavour.
3. Pour mixture into a pie or soufflé dish or dishes. Sprinkle with nutmeg.
4. Stand the baking dish(es) in a large baking dish. Carefully pour enough water into the large baking dish to reach two-thirds up the outside of the pie or soufflé dish(es).
5. Bake for 35 minutes if you are using individual dishes, 45 minutes if you are using one big dish. The custard should be lightly browned and set in the centre.

Nutrition data per serve: 266 kJ (63 cal), CHO 4 g, Protein 6 g, Fat 3 g.
Preparation time: 1 hour 10 minutes. Cooking equipment: deep pie or soufflé dish or four single-serve oven-proof dishes, large baking dish for water bath. Oven temperature: 150°C (300°F).

Dessert Ideas for Pancakes and Crêpes

Serves: 4

Crêpes Suzette
4 oranges, peeled and cut into segments, pith removed
juice of 1 orange
3 tbsp brandy
12 crêpes (recipe, page 82), warmed
garnish: rind of 1 orange, grated

Method:

1. Poach orange segments gently in orange juice until heated through.
2. Drain off juice and set aside.
3. Add brandy to fruit in frying pan, heat and ignite with a match or a lighter. Stir fruit gently and allow brandy to burn out.
5. Pour juice back into pan and reheat.
6. Place crêpes one by one in pan, filling each with fruit, and folding each into four to make a triangle. This allows crêpes to absorb the juice.
7. Serve topped with sprinkling of orange rind.

Nutrition data per serve: 992 kJ (237 cal), CHO 37 g, Protein 10 g, Fat 5 g.
Preparation time: 10 minutes. Cooking equipment: large frying pan.

Flambéed Pancakes or Crêpes

A mixture of fruits, for instance:

1 punnet strawberries, washed and hulled
2 bananas, sliced
8 apricots, stoned and quartered
juice of 1 orange
½ tsp ground cinnamon
4 tbsp brandy
8 Pancakes (recipe, page 83) or 12 Crêpes (recipe, page 82), warmed

Method:

1. In a frying pan, combine fruit and juice and simmer gently for approximately 5 minutes until fruit heats through and softens.
2. Drain off juice and set aside.
3. Add brandy to pan, heat and ignite with a match or lighter. Stir fruit gently and allow brandy to burn out.
4. Pour juice back into pan and reheat.
5. Divide fruit evenly between pancakes or crêpes and roll up or, if using crêpes, fold into four to make triangles.

Nutrition data per serve: 1236 kJ (296 cal), CHO 59 g, Protein 12 g, Fat 5 g.

Preparation time: 10 minutes. Cooking equipment: frying pan.

Berry and Cheese Pancakes

2 cups mixed berries, washed and hulled
1 tsp water
8 Pancakes (see recipe, page 83), warmed
8 tbsp cottage cheese

Method:

1. Poach berries in water for approximately 3 minutes until soft.
2. Divide fruit evenly between pancakes and top each with 1 tbsp cottage cheese.
3. Roll up and serve hot.

Nutrition dat per serve: 1158 kJ (266 cal), CHO 29 g, Protein 16 g, Fat 9 g.

Preparation time: 5 minutes. Cooking equipment: frying pan.

Apple and Sultana Pancakes

4 apples, peeled, cored and sliced
2 cloves
2 tbsp sultanas
8 Pancakes (recipe, page 83), warmed

Method:

1. Poach apples gently in a little water with cloves and sultanas for approximately 5 minutes until soft. Alternatively, microwave, covered, on 'high' for 5-8 minutes.
2. Remove cloves and divide apple mixture evenly between pancakes.
3. Roll up and serve hot.

Nutrition data per serve: 1183 kJ (283 cal), CHO 50 g, Protein 10 g, Fat 5 g.

Preparation time: 10 minutes. Cooking equipment: saucepan.

Buckwheat Pancakes with Blueberry Sauce

Makes 8 pancakes
(2 per serve)

½ cup buckwheat flour
½ cup plain flour
2 tsp baking powder
½ tsp cinnamon
1 tbsp sugar
1 egg, beaten
¾ cup low-fat milk
1 quantity Blueberry Sauce (recipe, page 165).

Method:

1. Sift flours, baking powder, and cinnamon into a mixing bowl. Return any husks to bowl.
2. Add sugar and mix in well.
3. Beat eggs and milk together.
4. Stir egg mixture slowly into the centre of the flour mixture, bringing flour in from the sides as you mix, then beat well until there are no lumps.
5. Heat frying pan, spraying with a little baking spray to prevent sticking.
6. Spoon 2 tbsp mixture into pan, cooking 2 pancakes at a time. When bubbles appear on the surface, turn the pancakes and cook on the other side until golden brown.
7. Keep warm until all pancakes are cooked.
8. Serve with blueberry sauce spooned over.

Nutrition data per serve: 691 kJ (165 cal), CHO 28 g, Protein 7.5 g, Fat 2.5 g.

Preparation time: 30 minutes. Cooking equipment: frying pan.

Rock Melon Sorbet with Blackcurrant or Raspberry Sauce

Serves: 4

Sorbet:

½ rock melon (cantaloupe)

juice of 1 lemon

1 sachet Equal™ or artificial sweetener equivalent to 2 tsp sugar

1 egg white, beaten until stiff

Sauce:

1 cup blackcurrants or 1½ cups raspberries, rinsed and hulled

¾-1 cup water

¼ tsp ground cinnamon

2 tsp cornflour (cornstarch)

1 tbsp water

1-2 sachet Equal™ or artificial sweetener equivalent to 2-4 tsp sugar

The key to a smooth sorbet is in the beating during the freezing process which ensures that the ice crystals which form are small and even.

Method:

Sorbet:
1. De-seed and peel rock melon (cantaloupe).
2. Cut into pieces and blend in food processor or blender until smooth.
3. Add lemon juice and Equal™ and blend again.
4. Pour into container, cover, and freeze for 2-3 hours until just set.
5. Reblend in food processor or blender or use an electric beater. The mixture should become creamy.
6. Fold in egg white.
7. Refreeze.
8. Before serving, remove sorbet from freezer and allow to soften a little.
9. Serve with sauce poured over.

Sauce:
10. Place berries, water and cinnamon in saucepan.
11. Heat gently until fruit has softened and lost its shape. Remove from heat.
12. Make a smooth paste of cornflour (cornstarch) and water and add to fruit, stirring well.
13. Reheat until mixture has thickened.
14. Cool, and add sweetener to taste.
15. Refrigerate until ready to serve.

Nutrition data per serve: 144 kJ (34 cal), CHO 7 g, Protein 2 g, Fat 0 g.

Preparation time: 1 hour. Cooking equipment: food processor, blender or electric beater, saucepan.

Golden Fruit Flummery

Serves: 12

1 pkt low-joule (low-calorie) jelly crystals, orange or orange and mango flavours
1½ cups boiling water
½ cup canned evaporated skim milk, chilled
400 g (13 oz) can solid packed unsweetened peach pieces, puréed
1 large mango puréed
garnish: Creamy Whipped Topping (recipe, page 165), sprig of mint

To prevent the evaporated milk separating from the rest of the flummery, you need to have the jelly and milk mixtures at approximately the same temperature before you combine them. Vary this recipe by a puréeing a 400 g (13 oz) can solid packed unsweetened apricot pieces instead of peaches and mango.

Method:

1. Dissolve jelly crystals in boiling water, cool, place in refrigerator until just beginning to set.
2. Whip jelly and, as it becomes fluffy, slowly add evaporated skim milk, whipping continually until the mixture thickens.
3. Gently mix in puréed fruit and pour into glass dishes.
4. Chill well before serving, garnished with a spoonful of whipped topping and a sprig of mint on each.

To store: cover and refrigerate for up to three days.

Nutrition data per serve: 131 kJ (31 cal), CHO 6 g, Protein 2 g, Fat trace.

Preparation time: 2 hours (including time taken to chill jelly).
Cooking equipment: electric beater.

Baked Yoghurt Slice

Serves: 8

Crust:
12 wheatmeal biscuits or 1 cup Meg's Muesli (recipe, page 58)
2-3 tbsp unsweetened apple juice
Filling:
1 cup low-fat fruit yoghurt
1¼ cups ricotta cheese
juice of 1 lemon

Method:

1. Grind the biscuits or muesli in food processor or blender or crush well with rolling pin.
2. Add apple juice to biscuit crumbs to make a spreadable mixture.
3. Line tart tin with aluminium foil.
4. Press the biscuit crumb mixture into lined tart tin.
5. Blend yoghurt, ricotta cheese, lemon juice and rind and apple juice in food processor or blender.
6. Beat egg whites stiffly.
7. Fold them through the blended cheese mixture with the sultanas.

rind of 1 lemon, grated
2 tbsp unsweetened apple juice
2 egg whites
½ cup sultanas

8. Pour into biscuit base.
9. Bake approximately 30 minutes until firm.
10. Cool and cut into slices.

To vary: use different flavoured yoghurt.

To store: cover with plastic film and refrigerate for up to two days.

Nutrition data per serve: 781 kJ (187 cal), CHO 25 g, Protein 8 g, Fat 6 g.
Preparation time: 1 hour. Cooking equipment: food processor, tart tin.
Oven temperature: 180°C (350°F).

Mocha Mousse

Serves: 4

2 eggs, separated
375 mL (13 fl oz) evaporated skim milk
1 tbsp cocoa
½ tsp instant coffee granules
3 tsp gelatine
3 tbsp water
3 sachets Equal™ or artificial sweetener equivalent to 6 tsp sugar
garnish: chopped dates or fresh strawberries

This is a scrumptious dessert. Prepare it the day before you want to serve it because it needs to set.

Method:

1. Beat egg yolks, and combine them in a saucepan with milk, cocoa and coffee. Mix until smooth.
2. Stirring constantly, warm the mixture over medium heat, being careful not to boil. Remove from heat and cool.
3. Sprinkle gelatine over water and dissolve over hot water, or microwave on 'medium' for 10 seconds. Cool slightly.
4. Stir into chocolate mixture. Add sweetener. Cool until mixture begins to set around edges.
5. Whip until thick and creamy.
6. Beat egg whites until soft peaks form. Fold into chocolate mixture.
7. Pour into serving dishes. Cover and refrigerate overnight.
8. Serve chilled and garnish with chopped dates or strawberries.

Nutrition data per serve: 169 kJ (40 cal), CHO 2 g, Protein 3 g, Fat 2 g.
Preparation time: 45 minutes, plus setting time. Cooking equipment: saucepan.

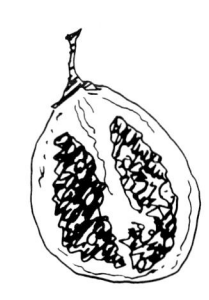

Bread and Butter Pudding

Serves: 4

4 eggs
600 mL (1 pint) skim or low-fat milk
2 tsp vanilla essence
3 slices wholemeal bread
2 tsp margarine
2 tbsp sultanas
1 tsp ground nutmeg

Method:

1. Place eggs in bowl and beat.
2. Add milk and vanilla essence.
3. Spread bread with margarine and cut each slice into four squares.
4. Place three squares in each individual baking dish.
5. Pour an equal amount of the mixture into each dish.
6. Sprinkle sultanas and nutmeg evenly into the four dishes.
7. Place the four individual dishes in a larger baking dish, and carefully pour water into the larger baking dish to reach two-thirds up the outside of the individual baking dishes.
8. Bake for 30-45 minutes until set, or arrange the puddings in a wide circle in the microwave to ensure even cooking. Microwave on 'medium' for 8-10 minutes.

Nutrition data per serve: 837 kJ (200 cal), CHO 19 g, Protein 13 g, Fat 8 g.
Preparation time: 1 hour. Cooking equipment: individual baking dishes, large baking dish for water bath. Oven temperature: 180°C (350°F).

[handwritten: Mark No 4]

Queen's Pudding

Serves: 4

4 eggs
600 mL (1 pint) skim or low-fat milk
2 tsp vanilla essence
3 slices wholemeal bread, crumbed
4 tbsp strawberry or raspberry purée
1 tbsp castor sugar

If you do not have any strawberry or raspberry purée, you can use low-joule (low-calorie) jam as a substitute.

Method:

1. Separate 2 eggs and put egg whites aside.
2. Combine egg yolks with other 2 whole eggs and beat.
3. Add milk and vanilla.
4. Distribute breadcrumbs evenly between four individual baking dishes.
5. Pour equal amounts of custard mixture into each dish.
6. Put individual dishes in a larger baking dish, and carefully pour in water until it reaches two-thirds up the outside of the individual baking dishes. Bake for 30-45 minutes.
7. When cooked, carefully spread top of custard with fruit purée.

Foreground left: Summer Pudding, at right Lemon and Cinnamon Cheese Cake, at centre left Apple Strudel, and Pumpkin Pie at top.

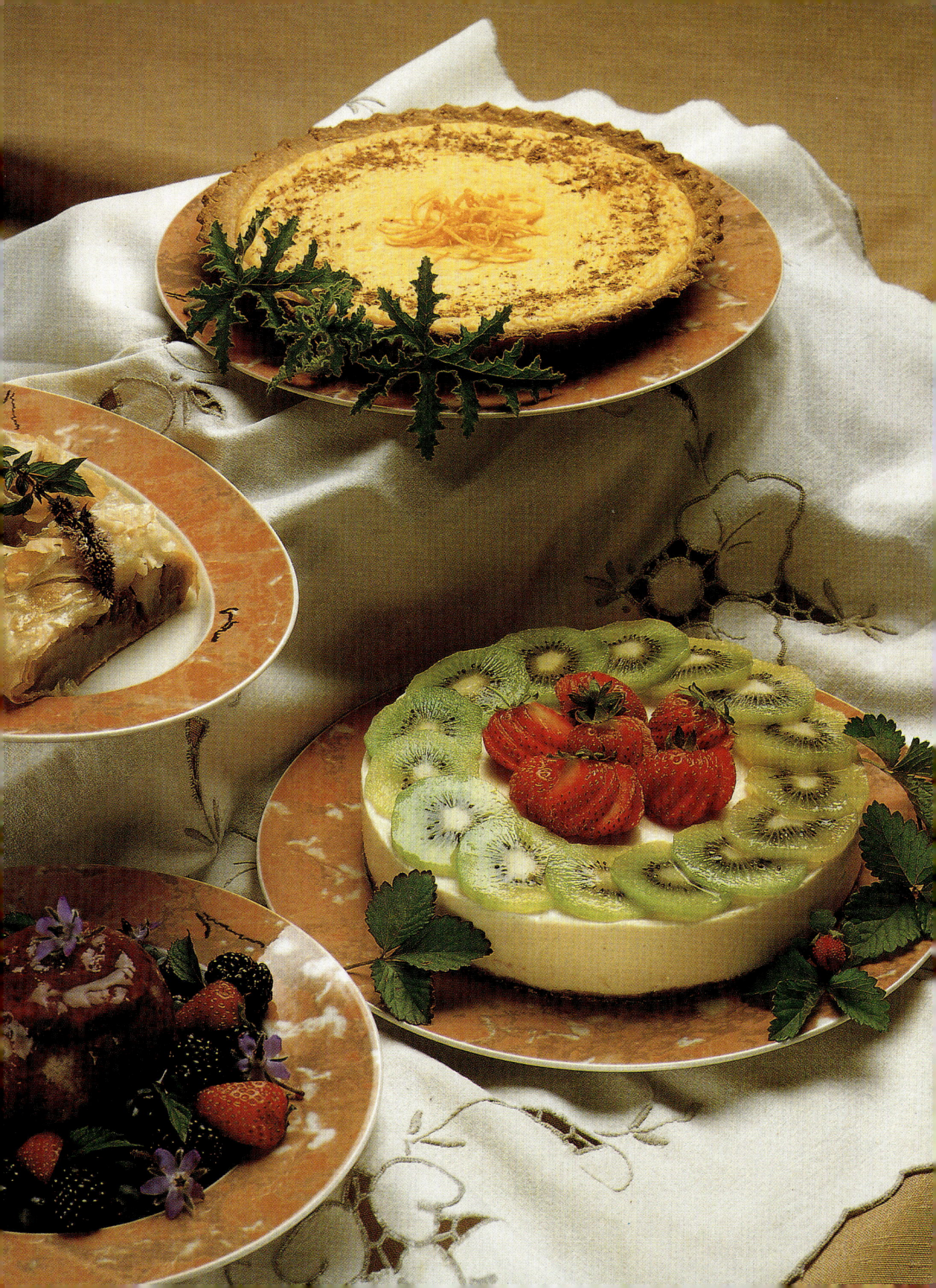

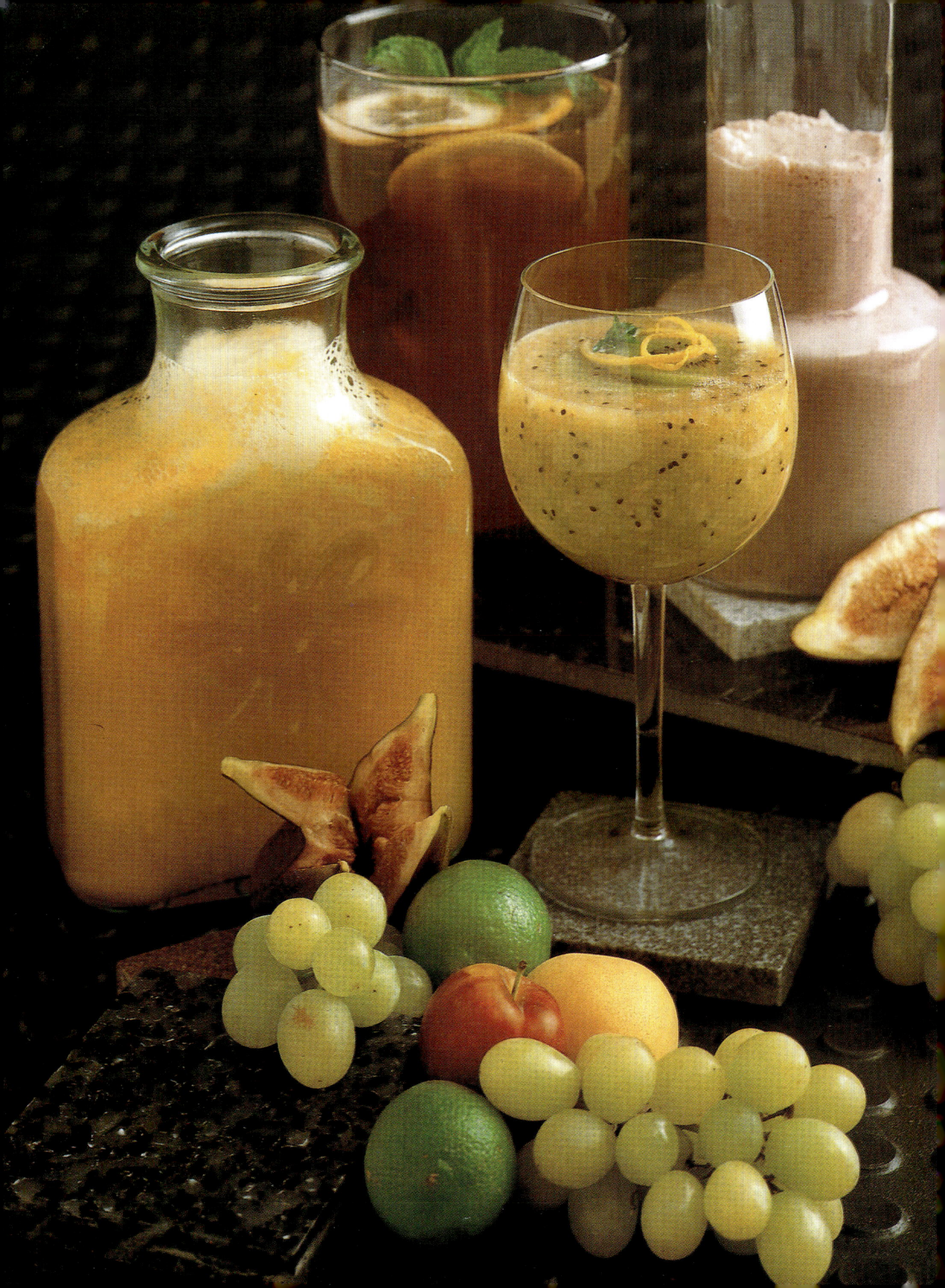

8. Beat the remaining 2 egg whites until they are stiff and fold in castor sugar and pile over purée.
9. Bake for about 5 minutes until meringue is lightly browned.

To store: cover and refrigerate for up to 2 days.

Nutrition data per serve: 793 kJ (189 cal), CHO 21 g, Protein 13 g, Fat 6 g.
Preparation time: 1½ hours. Cooking equipment: individual baking dishes, large baking dish for water bath. Oven temperature: 180°C (350°F).

Christmas Pudding

Serves: 6

4 tbsp sultanas
2 tbsp currants
3 tbsp raisins
rind of 1 orange, grated
½ cup grated carrot, apple or cooked pumpkin (or a mixture of two)
3 tbsp brandy
½ cup wholemeal flour
1 tsp ground cinnamon
1 tsp mixed spice
½ tsp nutmeg
2 tbsp margarine
1½ slices wholemeal bread, crumbed
1 egg, lightly beaten
⅓ cup skim or low-fat milk
1 tsp vanilla essence
2 tsp parisian essence
1 tbsp brown sugar or Sweetadin™
½ tsp bicarbonate of soda
1 tbsp hot water

This is better if made a week before you want to serve it, so that the flavours have time to mature.

Method:

1. Soak dried fruit, orange rind and carrot, apple or pumpkin in brandy overnight.
2. Mix flour and spices.
3. Rub margarine into flour mixture, and add breadcrumbs.
4. Add egg, milk, fruit mixture, vanilla, parisian essence and sugar or sweetener.
5. Combine bicarbonate of soda and hot water and mix well with other ingredients.
6. Pour into a greased bowl, cover securely and steam for 1½-2 hours.
7. Turn out and serve with Brandy Sauce (recipe, page 166).

To store: in refrigerator. Reheat by steaming or boiling for 30-45 minutes until heated through, or microwave, covered, on 'high' for 5-7 minutes. Do not store it again after you have reheated it.

Nutrition data per serve: 1246 kJ (298 cal), CHO 46 g, Protein 10 g, Fat 6 g.
Preparation time: 2½ hours, plus overnight.
Cooking equipment: pudding basin, steamer or large saucepan.

Front left: Apricot Cooler, in the glass (centre) Kiwi Cooler, top right, Cherries and Leben, top left, Sangria.

Eat & Enjoy   Desserts

Crunchy Peach Ice cream

Serves: 6-8

425 g (14 oz) can solid pack pie peaches
juice of ½ lemon
½ tsp ground cinnamon
50 g (1 oz) ricotta cheese
100 g (3 oz) low-fat natural yoghurt
Equal™ or 2 tbsp apple concentrate to taste
2 tsp liqueur (optional)
2 tbsp dessicated coconut
2 tbsp chopped blanched almonds, toasted
3 tbsp crunchy cereal (muesli, rice bubbles, etc)
1 egg white

The more carefully you beat the mixture part way through the freezing process, the smoother and creamier your ice cream will be. Homemade ice cream is better used fresh as ice cream tends to go hard if refrozen.

Method:

1. Blend fruit in food processor or blender until smooth and creamy.
2. Add other ingredients, blend well. Add liqueur if desired.
3. Spoon into container. Cover and freeze for 2-3 hours until almost set.
4. Remove and thaw slightly. Break up the ice crystals by returning to food processor or blender, blend until creamy, then spoon back into bowl and add coconut, nuts and cereal.
5. Beat egg white until soft peaks form.
6. Fold into ice cream, cover and refreeze until firm.
7. Remove and allow to thaw a little before serving as this ice cream is much more delicious if a little soft.

Nutrition data per serve: 348 kJ (83 cal), CHO 7 g, Protein 4 g, Fat 4 g.

Preparation time: 1 hour over 1-2 days. Cooking equipment: food processor or blender, mixing bowl with lid suitable for freezing.

Lemon and Cinnamon Cheesecake

Serves: 8

Biscuit base:
1 cup shredded wheatmeal biscuit crumbs
50 g (2 oz) almonds, crushed
1 tbsp margarine, melted
2 tsp water
2 tsp cinnamon
Filling:
300 mL (10 fl oz) buttermilk
250 g (8 oz) ricotta cheese
juice of 2 lemons
rind of 1 lemon, grated
1 tsp vanilla essence
1 tbsp sugar or Equal™ or other equivalent artificial sweetener
1 tbsp powdered gelatine
2 tbsp water
garnish:
  kiwifruit
  strawberries (optional)
  2 tsp cinnamon

You must make this recipe the day before you want to serve it to allow the filling to set.

Method:

Biscuit base:

1. Combine all ingredients for biscuit base.
2. Press mixture into a lined pie dish and refrigerate for 30 minutes.

Filling:

3. Mix buttermilk with ricotta cheese, lemon juice, lemon rind, vanilla essence and sugar or artificial sweetener. Beat until smooth and fluffly.
4. Dissolve gelatine in hot water. Cool slightly and fold into buttermilk mixture and blend well.
5. Pour into pie base and refrigerate until set.
6. Next day, decorate with sliced kiwifruit and a sprinkle of cinnamon.

To vary: replace lemons and lemon rind with the juice and rind of 1 orange.

To store: cover and refrigerate for up to three days.

Nutrition data per serve: 800 kJ (191 cal), CHO 14 g, Protein 7 g, Fat 12 g.

Preparation time: 1 hour, including chilling time for the base.
Cooking equipment: pie dish with removable base, electric beater.

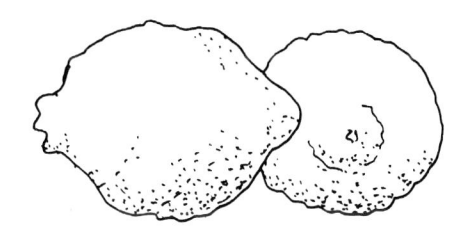

Baking

Herby Corn Muffins

Makes: 12

1 cup plain flour
1 cup cornmeal
½ tsp salt
2 tsp baking powder
1 tbsp margarine, melted
1 cup low-fat milk
1 egg, beaten
¼ tsp black pepper
½ tsp dried mixed herbs
2 tbsp grated low-fat block cheese

These savoury muffins are a great accompaniment to pumpkin or corn chowder. Eat them fresh because they won't keep.

Method:

1. Sift flours, salt and baking powder into a bowl.
2. Mix margarine, milk and egg and add to dry ingredients. Beat until smooth.
3. Fold in seasonings and cheese and spoon mixture into lightly greased muffin tins.
4. Bake for 15-20 minutes until golden brown. Turn out to cool.

Nutrition data per muffin: 471 kJ (112 cal), CHO 17 g, Protein 4 g, Fat 3 g.

Preparation time: 30 minutes. Cooking equipment: muffin tins. Oven temperature: 210°C (425°F).

Wholemeal Damper

Serves: 6

2 cups wholemeal self-raising flour
¼ tsp salt
2 tsp margarine
⅓ cup skim or low-fat milk
⅔ cup water
1 tbsp sesame seeds

Method:

1. Sift flour into mixing bowl. Return bran to sifted flour.
2. Rub margarine into flour until mixture resembles fine breadcrumbs.
3. Combine milk and water, and pour into dry ingredients. Mix quickly, blending with a knife.
4. Turn onto a floured board. Work into a round shape.
5. Place on lightly greased baking tray. Sprinkle with sesame seeds. Bake for 20-30 minutes until brown. Eat while warm.

Nutrition data per serve: 767 kJ (183 cal), CHO 31 g, Protein 7 g, Fat 3 g.

Preparation time: 50 minutes. Cooking equipment: baking tray. Oven temperature: 220°C (440°F).

Banana Muffins

Makes: 12

2 very ripe bananas
1 egg
½ cup skim or low-fat milk
½ cup unsweetened apple juice
1 cup wholemeal self-raising flour
1 cup white self-raising flour
½ tsp ground cinnamon
½ tsp baking powder

Muffins for breakfast, muffins for school lunch, muffins as a snack . . . muffins full of carbohydrate and fibre.

Method:

1. Mash bananas very well. There should be no lumps.
2. Beat egg and add to banana.
3. Add milk and apple juice.
4. Sift flours, cinnamon and baking powder.
5. Fold flours into liquid mixture. Mix well by hand.
6. Spoon into very lightly greased muffin tins, filling each up by about two thirds.
7. Bake for about 20 minutes until lightly browned and cooked through. Remove from oven, lift muffins out of tins and cool on a cake rack.

Nutrition data per muffin: 468 kJ (112 cal), CHO 21 g, Protein 4 g, Fat 1 g.
Preparation time: 40 minutes. Cooking equipment: muffin tin. Oven temperature: 210°C (425°F).

Mark 7

Chris's Cookies

Makes: 24 cookies

1 cup rolled oats
1 cup wholemeal self-raising flour
½ cup rice bran or oat bran
½ cup Splenda™ (or equivalent granulated sweetener)
½ cup desiccated coconut
½ cup currants
2 large very ripe bananas, mashed
2 eggs, beaten

You can use sultanas or chopped dried apricots instead of currants to make these quick and easy cookies.

Method:

1. Mix dry ingredients, add banana and eggs and mix well.
2. Break off small pieces and roll into balls, place on lightly greased oven trays, flatten each ball with the back of a fork.
3. Bake for about 15 minutes or until just beginning to brown.
4. Remove from oven trays, and cool on cake rack.

Nutrition data per cookie: 489 kJ (117 cal), CHO 18 g, Protein 4 g, Fat 3 g.
Preparation time: 25 minutes. Cooking equipment: 2 oven trays. Oven temperature: 180°C (350°F).

Mark 4

Eat & Enjoy — Baking

Wholemeal Pastry

1 cup wholemeal flour
1 cup plain flour
120 g (4 oz) margarine
juice of ½ lemon
½–¾ cup of iced water

You can use 2 cups of wholemeal flour if you like, but the pastry will be heavier than the version we suggest here. A food processor is a great help; it turns pastry-making into a quick and easy process, but be careful not to over-process the pastry or it will become heavy.

Method:

1. Combine the flours in a large bowl.
2. Rub the margarine into the flour until the mixture resembles breadcrumbs.
3. Combine juice and water and add it to the dry ingredients, a little at a time, working it in after each addition, until you have a soft dough.
4. Turn dough onto a lightly floured board and knead lightly. Cover and allow to rest before using.
5. Use dough as required.

Note: Most pastries need to be baked in a hot oven — 200°C (400°F) — for 15 minutes, or until lightly browned.

To store: wrap in plastic film and refrigerate for up to two days.

Nutrition data per quantity: 7831 kJ (1871 cal), CHO 193 g, Protein 36 g, Fat 104 g.
Preparation time: 15 minutes. Oven temperature: 200°C (400°F).

No. 6

Pikelets

Makes: 12-16

¾ cup self-raising flour
¾ cup wholemeal self-raising flour
1 egg
¾ cup skim or low-fat milk
a little oil for frying

We have given special recipes for conserves and spreads in this book; they are perfect served with these pikelets.

Method:

1. Place flour in basin and make a well in the centre.
2. Beat egg and mix in milk in a small bowl.
3. Pour the egg and milk mixture into the centre of the flour and gradually beat in the flour using a wooden spoon.
4. Beat mixture well.
5. Heat frying pan and lightly oil.
6. Drop spoonfuls of mixture into pan allowing room for each pikelet to spread.

7. When mixture begins to bubble, turn over with a knife or egg slice.
8. Let pikelets cook until light brown on each side and lift onto a clean cloth. Keep covered with cloth to keep them soft.
9. Serve with Fresh Strawberry Conserve (recipe, page 59), Dried Apricot Conserve (recipe, page 60) or Date and Fig Spread (recipe, page 60).

Nutrition data per pikelet (if 12 made): 341 kJ (81 cal), CHO 13 g, Protein 3 g, Fat 2 g.
Preparation time: 30 minutes. Cooking equipment: large frying pan.

Quick Wholemeal Bread

Makes: 2 loaves, each of 18 slices

4 cups wholemeal flour
2 tsp bicarbonate of soda
500 mL (17 fl oz) full-cream natural yoghurt
1 tbsp honey (optional)
topping: 1 tbsp sesame seeds (optional)

This quick and easy loaf contains no yeast, so there is no kneading and rising time required. You can vary the recipe by adding half a cup of roughly chopped pecan nuts or walnuts. Alternatively, try adding half a cup of sunflower seeds or raisins. You may prefer the flavour of the loaf with the addition of a little salt at Step 3, but try it without first.

Method:
1. Lightly grease the loaf tin.
2. Measure the flour, unsifted, into a large bowl.
3. Add all remaining ingredients, except the sesame seeds. Use a wooden spoon to mix lightly but well, until mixture is fluffy.
4. Spoon mixture into the greased loaf tin. Sprinkle with sesame seeds.
5. Bake for 50-60 minutes, or until loaf sounds hollow when tapped.

To store: keep in an airtight container for up to two days.

Nutrition data per slice: 280 kJ (67 cal), CHO 11 g, Protein 3 g, Fat 1 g.
Preparation time: approximately 1 hour. Cooking equipment: 2 loaf tins. Oven temperature: 180°C (350°F).

Mark no. 4

Eat & Enjoy   *Baking*   191

Carrot Cake

Makes: 20 slices

2 cups wholemeal self-raising flour *[250 gr]*
½ tsp bicarbonate of soda
2 tsp ground cinnamon
1 tsp ground nutmeg
1 tsp mixed spice
2 cups grated carrot *[200 gr]*
½ cup shredded coconut *[50 gr]*
½ cup chopped walnuts *[75 g]*
½ cup sultanas *[75 gr]*
2 eggs
¼ cup apple concentrate
1 cup skim or low-fat milk *[¼ pt]*

Method:

1. Grease and lightly flour cake tin.
2. Sift flour, soda and spices. Return bran to flour mixture.
3. Add carrot, coconut, nuts and sultanas.
4. Beat eggs until fluffy and add apple concentrate. Beat again and add milk.
5. Fold into dry ingredients. Stir until well mixed and pour batter into prepared cake tin.
6. Bake until cooked through (approximately 40-45 minutes).
7. Turn out and cool on cake rack.

To vary: replace walnuts with pecans.

To store: keep in an airtight container for up to four days.

Nutrition data per slice: 475 kJ (113 cal), CHO 16 g, Protein 4 g, Fat 4 g.

Preparation time: 1 hour. Cooking equipment: 20 cm (8 in) cake tin. Oven temperature: 200°C (400°F).

Scones

Makes: 12

1 cup wholemeal self-raising flour
1 cup self-raising flour, less 1 heaped tbsp
1 heaped tbsp gluten flour
½ tsp baking powder
1 tbsp margarine
½ cup low-fat milk
½ cup low-fat natural yoghurt

Gluten flour used in this recipe is available from health food shops and some supermarkets. The key to perfect scones is to handle the dough quickly and lightly so that it keeps plenty of air in it, and to bake them in a hot oven.

Method:

1. In a bowl, combine the flours and baking powder. Use your fingertips to rub the margarine into the dry ingredients until the mixture resembles fine breadcrumbs.
2. Add the milk and yoghurt. Use a knife to work the mixture until you have a fine soft dough.
3. Turn the dough onto a lightly floured board. Using your finger tips quickly and lightly knead the dough until soft and smooth.

4. Gently flatten the dough to a 2 cm (¾ in) thickness.
5. Use a scone cutter or sharp knife to shape 12 scones. Avoid rerolling and cutting dough scraps more than once.
6. Place the scones on a lightly greased baking tray. Leave a gap about half the width of a scone between each one.
7. If you want the scones to brown on top, brush each one with a little milk and bake them near the top of the oven.
8. Bake for 8-10 minutes.

Nutrition data per scone: 454 kJ (108 cal), CHO 17 g, Protein 4 g, Fat 2 g.
Preparation time: 20 minutes. Cooking equipment: baking tray.
Oven temperature: 220°C (440°F).

Fruit Scones   Knead 2 tablespoons of sultanas, currants or chopped dates into the dough mixture at Step 2.

Bluestone Muffins

Makes: 12

1 cup ripe blueberries
4 tsp brown sugar
2 cups wholemeal self-raising flour
1 tsp baking powder
1 tsp ground cinnamon
1 egg
½ cup low-fat berry yoghurt
1 cup skim or low-fat milk

They look a little strange, perhaps, but taste terrific. Eat them fresh; they won't keep. Remember, a trace of sugar will not harm you, particularly when combined with plenty of complex carbohydrate and fibre.

Method:

1. Lightly grease muffin tins or spray with cooking spray.
2. Wash blueberries and combine with sugar in saucepan.
3. Heat gently until juice just starts to run.
4. Sift flour, baking powder and cinnamon into bowl. Return bran to flour mixture.
5. Mix egg, yoghurt and milk in a bowl. Add to flour and blend until smooth.
6. Gently fold blueberries into mixture.
7. Spoon mixture into muffin tins, and bake for 15-20 minutes until firm and very lightly browned.

Nutrition data per muffin: 486 kJ (116 cal), CHO 21 g, Protein 5 g, Fat 1 g.
Preparation time: 40 minutes. Cooking equipment: saucepan, muffin tins.
Oven temperature: 210°C (425°F).

Fruit (Christmas) Cake

Makes: 24 slices

1½ cups sultanas
½ cup raisins, chopped
2 tbsp brandy
1 tbsp water
1 cup sieved pumpkin (no lumps)
2 eggs, beaten
½ cup apple concentrate
½ cup skim or low-fat milk
½ cup chopped pecans
1 tsp ground cinnamon
1 tsp mixed spice
1 cup white self-raising flour
1 cup wholemeal self-raising flour
½ tsp bicarbonate of soda

Apple concentrate gives sweetness to this wonderful fruity cake, and the dried fruit and pumpkin add plenty of fibre.

Method:

1. Mix sultanas, raisins, brandy and water, soak overnight.
2. Mix pumpkin, eggs, apple concentrate and milk.
3. Add soaked fruit, nuts and spices, then sifted flour and bicarbonate of soda. Return bran left in sieve to flour mixture. Mix well with a wooden spoon.
4. Spoon into a lightly greased cake tin.
5. Bake 10 minutes at 200°C (400°F), then turn down the heat and bake at 180°C (350°F) until cooked through and browned (approximately 1-1¼ hours). Cool on a cake rack.

To store: keep in an airtight container for up to 1 week.

Nutrition data per slice: 482 kJ (115 cal), CHO 21 g, Protein 3 g, Fat 2 g.

Preparation time: 1½ hours, plus overnight soaking.
Cooking equipment: round or square cake tin 20 cm (8 in).
Oven temperature: 200°C (400°F), then 180°C (350°F).

Mince Tarts

Makes: 12

Filling:
½ cup chopped dried apricots
1 cup sultanas
½ cup chopped pitted dates
12 prunes, seeded and chopped
6 dried figs, chopped
½ cup slivered almonds

You can store any extra filling in a closed jar in the refrigerator for up to two weeks.

Method:

Filling:

1. Combine all ingredients in saucepan.
2. Cook, covered, over low heat until apple is soft. Stir frequently to prevent sticking.
3. Spoon into bowl, cover and refrigerate overnight to blend flavours.

2 apples, peeled, cored
   and thinly sliced
juice of ½ lemon
½ cup brandy
½ tsp cinnamon
½ tsp ground nutmeg
½ tsp mixed spice

Pastry:
½ cup wholemeal flour
1 cup plain flour
4 tbsp margarine
2-3 tbsp iced water
1 egg yolk
few drops liquid
   artificial sweetener

Pastry:

4. Sift flours into bowl, return bran left in sieve to sifted flour.
5. Rub margarine into flour until mixture resembles breadcrumbs.
6. In a cup combine water, egg yolk and sweetener.
7. Add to flour mixture and stir in with a knife. Turn out onto floured board. Knead lightly, then cover and leave to rest for 10-15 minutes.
8. Roll out dough and cut 12 rounds to fit the bottom of the tart tins. Cut another 12, slightly smaller, to make the lids.
9. Lightly grease the tart tins and line the bases.
10. Spoon some fruit mince into each.
11. Wet pastry edges and place remaining pastry rounds on top. Pinch edges to seal. Prick tops with fork.
12. Bake for 20-30 minutes until lightly browned.

Nutrition data per tart: 1130 kJ (270 cal), CHO 43 g, Protein 5 g, Fat 9 g.

Preparation time: 1½ hours, plus overnight soaking.
Cooking equipment: saucepan, tart tins.
Oven temperature: 190°C (375°F).

Apple and Apricot Slice

Makes: 16 pieces

1 quantity Wholemeal
   Pastry (recipe, page 190)
500 g (1 lb) fresh
   apricots, stoned and
   quartered or 400 g
   (13 oz) can
   unsweetened
   apricot pieces
3 apples, peeled, cored
   and thinly sliced
½ tsp cinnamon
skim milk for glazing

Method:

1. Divide pastry into two equal pieces. Roll out first half and cover base of lightly greased biscuit tray.
2. Mix fruit and cinnamon and spread evenly on pastry.
3. Roll second half of pastry and place over fruit.
4. Prick surface of pastry with fork or skewer, brush with milk and bake for 30 minutes or until pastry is beginning to brown.
5. Stand on cake rack for 5 minutes, loosen around the edges and turn out. Cool and cut into 16 even pieces.

Nutrition data per piece: 569 kJ (136 cal), CHO 17 g, Protein 3 g, Fat 7 g.

Preparation time: 50 minutes.
Cooking equipment: biscuit tray, 28 cm x 19 cm (12 in x 8 in).
Oven temperature: 200°C (400°F).

Date and Walnut Loaf

Makes: 10 slices

½ cup boiling water
1 cup chopped dates
1½ cups wholemeal self-raising flour
1 tsp mixed spice
1 tsp ground cinnamon
2 tbsp margarine
1 tbsp sugar
½ cup chopped walnuts
1 egg, beaten
1 cup skim milk

Don't limit yourself to dates and walnuts; substitute any other dried fruit and nuts you choose.

Method:

1. Pour boiling water over dates and let stand for 30 minutes.
2. Mix flour and spices in bowl.
3. Rub in margarine until mixture resembles breadcrumbs.
4. Add sugar, dates, soaking water and walnuts to dry mixture and mix lightly.
5. Stir in egg and skim milk.
6. Place in lightly greased nut loaf tin.
7. Bake upright for 45 minutes or until cooked.
8. Leave in tin for 10 minutes before turning out to cool.

Nutrition data per slice: 976 kJ (233 cal), CHO 35 g, Protein 6 g, Fat 8 g.
Preparation time: 1 hour and 10 minutes. Cooking equipment: nut loaf tin. Oven temperature: 190°C (375°F) for 20 minutes, then lower to 180°C (350°F) for a further 25 minutes.

Wholemeal Apple-nut Streusel Cake

Serves: 16 slices

150 g (5 oz) margarine
¾ cup Splenda™ (or equivalent granulated sweetener)
100 g (3 oz) ricotta cheese
1 tsp vanilla essence
3 eggs
½ cup white self-raising flour
1½ cup wholemeal plain flour
1 tsp bicarbonate of soda
1 cup skim milk
1 apple, peeled and grated
¾ cup sultanas
1 cup chopped pecans or walnuts
½ tsp ground cinnamon

Method:

1. Lightly grease and line the base of cake tin.
2. Cream margarine and Splenda, then beat in ricotta and essence.
3. Add eggs one at a time and beat in.
4. Mix flours and soda and fold into mixture with milk.
5. Add apple and sultanas and mix.
6. Spread ½ mixture into cake tin. Sprinkle over ½ nuts and cinnamon. Spread with remaining cake mixture and sprinkle with remaining nuts and cinnamon.
7. Bake for 1 hour or until cooked.
8. Cool slightly before turning out.

To store: Cover and refrigerate for up to four days.

Nutrition data per slice: 807 kJ (193 cal), CHO 15 g, Protein 5 g, Fat 13 g.
Preparation time: 1¼ hours. Cooking equipment: 20 cm (8 in) cake tin. Oven temperature: 180°C (350°F).

After-Dinner Treats

Date Rolls

Makes: 20 pieces

2 cups seeded dates
juice of 1 lemon
½ tsp ground cinnamon
½ cup roasted hazelnuts, crushed
4 tbsp poppy seeds
4 shredded wheatmeal biscuits, crushed

Method:

1. Blend dates with lemon juice and cinnamon to a thick paste.
2. Add nuts and poppy seeds, and mix well.
3. Form into four rolls, each approximately 10 cm (4 in) long and 2½ cm (1 in) thick. Roll in crushed wheatmeal biscuits.
4. Refrigerate for 2 hours, and then cut each roll into five equal pieces approximately 2 cm (¾ in) thick.

Nutrition data per piece: 313 kJ (75 cal), CHO 13 g, Protein 2 g, Fat 2 g.

Preparation time: 30 minutes. Equipment: food processor or blender.

Fruit Cheese

Makes: 1 log approximately 20 cm (8 in) long

½ cup dried fruit medley
½ cup hot water
3 tbsp brandy
125 g (4 oz) each of cottage cheese and cream cheese or 250 g (8 oz) low-fat cream cheese
3 tbsp poppy seeds

This after-dinner treat can be made one or two days before serving and then be stored in the refrigerator until needed.

Method:

1. Place fruit in bowl and pour over water and brandy. Allow to soak for about 12 hours until fruit is swollen and soft.
2. Drain fruit, retaining the liquid.
3. Blend cheese and ¼ cup of the drained liquid until smooth. Discard remaining drained liquid.
4. Stir fruit into mixture and mix well.
5. Tip mixture onto plastic film. Form into a rough log shape. Roll plastic film around log and refrigerate for 1 hour to set.
6. Spread poppy seeds over a clean piece of plastic film and roll cheese log on this to coat with seeds. Return to refrigerator for two hours before serving.

To store: cover and refrigerate for up to four days.

Nutrition data per total quantity: 4221 kJ (1008 cal), CHO 72 g, Protein 45 g, Fat 47 g.
Preparation time: 10 minutes, plus 12 hours soaking time and 3 hours setting time.

Rum Balls

Makes: 24

20 shredded wheatmeal biscuits
8 tsp cocoa
150 g (5 oz) ricotta cheese
3 tbsp unsweetened apple juice
2 tbsp brown rum
½ tsp vanilla essence (optional)
1 cup desiccated coconut

Method:

1. Process biscuits in food processor or blender until they resemble fine crumbs.
2. Add cocoa, ricotta cheese, apple juice, rum and vanilla and blend well.
3. Spoon into a mixing bowl, cover and refrigerate overnight.
4. Roll a small spoonful of mixture in coconut, place on tray and refrigerate.

To vary: add ¼ cup chopped raisins.

To store: keep in airtight container for up to a week.

Nutrition data per ball: 327 kJ (78 cal), CHO 8 g, Protein 2 g, Fat 4 g.

Preparation time: 30 minutes, spread over two days, plus overnight. Equipment: food processor or blender.

Frozen Fruit

Serves: 4

8 strawberries, tops left on
20 purple grapes, preferably small
½ slice fresh ripe pineapple
2 kiwifruit
garnish: mint, ivy or strawberry leaves

We have used fresh strawberries, grapes, pineapple and kiwifruit in this recipe, but you can use any selection of fresh fruit in season. You can also use frozen fruit to garnish drinks.

Method:

1. Wash and dry strawberries and grapes.
2. Cut pineapple into eight chunks.
3. Peel kiwifruit and cut into four pieces.
4. Place fruit on shallow dish and freeze for approximately two hours until firm.
5. Transfer frozen fruit to glass serving plate, and allow to thaw for 10-15 minutes. Decorate with leaves.

To store: sealed, in freezer, if it is to be kept more than 24 hours.

Nutrition data per serve: 123 kJ (30 cal), CHO 7 g, Protein 1 g, Fat 0 g.

Preparation time: 2½ hours. Equipment: tray or shallow dish.

Drinks

50/50 Swirl
Serves: 4

For special occasions, use chilled champagne instead of bitter lemon.

Pour 2 cups unsweetened orange juice into a shallow tray and freeze until almost set. Crush and spoon into 4 chilled glasses. Pour half a 285 mL (10 fl oz) bottle of low-joule (low-calorie) bitter lemon into each glass and add a swirl of lemon and orange peel.

Nutrition data per serve: 175 kJ (42 cal), CHO 9 g, Protein 1 g, Fat 0 g.

Orange Buttermilk
Serves: 4

Place 1½ cups buttermilk in a jug, then slowly add 1½ cups unsweetened orange juice, stirring constantly. Sweeten with Equal™ or other artificial sweetener if desired, and pour into glasses, garnished with ice-cubes.

Nutrition data per serve: 262 kJ (63 cal), CHO 11 g, Protein 4 g, Fat 0 g.

Strawberry Granita
Serves: 2

Wash and hull a punnet of strawberries and add to food processor or blender with 8-10 ice-cubes and the juice of an orange. Blend until ice is crushed. Add Equal™ or other artificial sweetener to taste, then quickly blend again. Pour into glasses.

Nutrition data per serve: 164 kJ (39 cal), CHO 7 g, Protein 2 g, Fat 0 g.

Irish Coffee
Serves: 4

Bring ½ cup whisky to the boil and simmer for 30 seconds (or microwave on 'high' for 1 minute). Pour into each of four cups, top with hot black coffee and a tablespoon of Creamy Whipped Topping (recipe, page 165). Sweeten to taste with Equal™ or other artificial sweetener.

Nutrition data per serve: 43 kJ (10 cal), CHO 2 g, Protein 1 g, Fat 0 g.

Apricot Cooler
Serves: 4

Place 1 can (425 g/14 oz) solid pack unsweetened apricot pieces and ½ cup unsweetened apricot nectar or orange juice in a food processor or blender. Blend until smooth. Chill well, then pour into four glasses. Top with soda water. Garnish with mint.

Nutrition data per serve: 183 kJ (44 cal), CHO 11 g, Protein 1 g, Fat 0 g.

Sangria

Serves: 4

Bring 2 cups claret and ½ cup water to the boil in a saucepan and simmer for 30 seconds. Thinly slice 1 orange and 1 lemon and place in a jug. Pour wine over the lemon and orange slices and marinate in the refrigerator for 4 hours. Strain the mixture, add ½ cup unsweetened orange juice, sweeten to taste with Equal™ or other artificial sweetener, and serve with two ice-blocks and an orange slice.

Nutrition data per serve: 46 kJ (11 cal), CHO 2 g, Protein 0 g, Fat 0 g.

Hot Claret Punch

Serves: 4

Combine 2½ cups claret, 3 tbsps brandy in a saucepan or microwave dish. Bring to boil and simmer for 30 seconds, or microwave on 'high' for 4 minutes. Sweeten to taste with Equal™ or other artificial sweetener, pour into glasses and sprinkle with nutmeg.

Nutrition data per serve: 22 kJ (5 cal), CHO 1 g, Protein 0 g, Fat 0 g.

Cherries and Leben

Serves: 2

Place ½ cup pitted fresh cherries in a food processor or blender and blend until smooth. Add 1½ cups leben (or ¾ cup low-fat milk and ¾ cup low fat natural yoghurt), ¼ tsp ground cinnamon, a sachet of Equal™ or other artificial sweetener equivalent to 2 tsps sugar, and 4-6 ice-cubes. Blend again until thoroughly combined. Pour into glasses and serve.

Nutrition data per serve: 551 kJ (132 cal), CHO 17 g, Protein 10 g, Fat 3 g.

Kiwi Cooler

Serves: 4

Peel 4 kiwifruit and add to food processor or blender with 2 peeled and stoned peaches, 2 peeled and chopped bananas, 2 cups unsweetened pineapple juice and 8-10 ice-cubes. Blend until ice is crushed. Pour into glasses and garnish with a sprig of mint.

Nutrition data per serve: 539 kJ (129 cal), CHO 30 g, Protein 2 g, Fat 0 g.

Hot Milk Sleeper

Serves: 1

Separate an egg, beat the white until stiff and beat the yolk separately with 30 mL (1 fl oz) brandy and 1 tsp vanilla essence. Heat 200 mL (7 fl oz) skim or low-fat milk and add to egg yolk mixture. Fold in egg white, sweeten to taste with Equal™ or other artificial sweetener, pour into a large mug, sprinkle with nutmeg and serve.

Nutrition data per serve: 859 kJ (205 cal), CHO 10 g, Protein 13 g, Fat 5 g.

THE DETAILED FOOD VALUE LIST

We have included this food value chart to help you find out more about food and what's in it. It is not an essential part of your diabetes management, but you may find it interesting and useful. Most people use a limited range of food in their day-to-day eating pattern. This list may give you the confidence to include a wider variety of food when eating at home or out.

We have given the quantity of foods as 'average serves' to give you a measuring stick for the amount of energy, carbohydrate, protein and fat in different food items. It will allow you to compare foods, and immediately identify those foods high or low in carbohydrate, protein or fat.

The tables show the most up-to-date figures available, and are based on information supplied by the Department of Health.

Foods vary greatly in their nutrition content, depending on such things as place of origin, ripeness and season. In view of this, we have rounded off all figures to the nearest whole number. So use the chart as a guide only to nutrition values.

Foods have been arranged according to food groups and preferred choices are listed first (that is higher fibre or lower fat) where appropriate, or otherwise listed alphabetically.

Food Measure	Serve	g	Energy kJ	cal	C g	P g	F g
BREADS							
Wholemeal/multigrain	1 slice	30	271	65	12	3	1
Rye/black	1 slice	50	424	101	19	4	1
Fibre increased	1 slice	30	270	67	12	3	1
White	1 slice	30	291	70	13	2	1
Raisin	1 slice	30	329	79	16	2	1
Bread roll, wholemeal	1 small	60	600	143	26	6	1
Bread roll, white	1 small	60	649	155	29	6	2
Muffin	1 whole	70	640	153	29	6	1
Crumpet	1 med	40	314	75	16	2	neg
Bagel	1 med	80	720	179	32	8	3
Matzos	1	23	288	69	14	2	1
Flatbread/pocket/pita	1 large	100	1122	268	52	9	2
	1 small	60	673	161	31	5	1
Breadcrumbs, dried	2 tbsp	20	302	72	14	2	1
BISCUITS							
Ryvita™	2	20	301	72	16	2	1
Krispy Wheat™/ Sesawheat™	4	20	384	92	14	2	3
Vitawheat™	4	28	480	112	20	2	3
Rye Cruskits™	4	20	306	73	15	3	1
Salada, wholemeal™	4 small	14	240	56	10	2	1
Salada, plain™	4 small	16	260	64	11	2	2
Uneeda™	4	22	400	94	16	2	3
Thin Captains™	4	22	380	92	17	3	2
Crackerbread™	4	28	482	115	19	4	3
Sao™	2	18	329	79	12	2	3
Savoy™	6	25	470	113	17	2	5
Shredded Wheat™	2	16	270	64	11	1	2
Morning Coffee™	2	16	290	68	13	1	2
Marie	2	16	300	70	13	1	2
Gingernuts	2	27	470	112	23	1	2
BREAKFAST CEREALS							
Wheatgerm	2 tbsp	10	128	30	4	3	1
All-bran	1/2 cup	20	231	55	8	3	1
Rolled oats, raw	1/3 cup	35	568	136	25	5	3
Rolled oats, cooked	1 cup	260	551	132	22	4	3
Oat bran, raw	1 tbsp	11	113	27	7	2	1
Wheat flake biscuits, e.g., Weetbix™, Vitabrits™	2	30	398	95	19	3	neg
Muesli, unsweetened, untoasted	1/2 cup	55	846	202	31	7	5
Wheat flakes, e.g., Weeties™	1 cup	30	452	108	22	4	neg
Bran Flakes™	1 cup	45	618	148	28	6	1
Puffed Wheat™	1 cup	12	182	43	9	2	neg
Cornflakes™	1 cup	30	465	111	26	3	neg
Rice Bubbles™	1 cup	30	444	106	25	2	neg

*C = Carbohydrate   P = Protein   F = Fat   A = Alcohol   neg = negligible

Eat & Enjoy   *Food Lists*

Food Measure	Serve	g	Energy kJ	cal	C g	P g	F g	Food Measure	Serve	g	Energy kJ	cal	C g	P g	F g
FLOUR AND OTHER CEREALS								Artichoke, glob							
Buckwheat groats, raw	1/2 cup	50	760	182	42	4	0	Asparagus							
Cracked wheat/ kibbled wheat/ bulgar/burghul, dry	1/4 cup	45	563	134	27	5	1	Bean shoots/sprouts							
								Beans, french							
								Beetroot							
Flour, wholemeal	2 tbsp	20	235	56	10	2	neg	Broad beans							
Flour, white	2 tbsp	20	295	70	15	2	neg	Broccoli							
Cornflour	2 tbsp	20	312	75	20	neg	0	Brussels sprouts							
Pearl barley	2 tbsp	35	446	107	21	3	1	Cabbage							
Rice, brown, raw	3 tbsp	60	919	220	46	5	1	Capsicum (bell pepper)							
Rice, brown, cooked	1 cup	180	1134	271	57	6	2	Carrot							
Rice, white, raw	3 tbsp	60	885	211	48	4	neg	Cauliflower							
Rice, white, cooked	1 cup	190	993	237	53	4	neg	Celery							
Pasta, macaroni, spaghetti, raw		100	1426	341	70	11	1	Chinese cabbage							
								Choko							
Pasta, macaroni, spaghetti, cooked	1 cup	140	699	167	34	6	neg	Cucumber							
								Eggplant (aubergine)							
Egg pasta, cooked	1 cup	200	1093	261	51	10	1	Endive							
Sago, dry	2 tbsp	20	300	72	18	neg	0	Garlic							
Semolina, dry	2 tbsp	20	300	72	16	2	neg								
Custard powder	2 tbsp	20	292	70	17	neg	0	**FRUIT, edible portion**							
PULSES								Apple, fresh	1 med	120	235	56	14	0	0
Dried beans (borlotti, white, black-eyed, etc.), uncooked	1 tbsp	25	290	69	10	6	neg	Apple, canned/stewed	1 cup	240	237	79	20	0	0
								Apple juice	1/2 cup	120	170	41	10	0	0
cooked	1/2 cup	90	375	84	17	6	neg	Apricot, fresh	3 med	90	105	25	6	1	0
Baked beans, canned with tomato sauce	1/2 cup	120	324	77	12	6	1	Apricot, canned/stewed	1 cup	230	228	55	12	2	0
Mixed bean salad, canned	1/2 cup	100	446	106	17	6	1	Apricot, dried	10 hlvs	40	310	74	17	2	0
								Avocado	1/4 med	75	659	157	0	1	17
Chick peas, uncooked	1 tbsp	25	339	81	11	5	neg	Banana	1 med	100	384	92	21	2	0
cooked	1 cup	160	848	203	28	13	neg	Berries, blackberry, raspberry	1 cup	133	140	33	7	1	0
Lentils, uncooked	1 tbsp	25	352	84	15	6	neg	Berries, blueberry	1 cup	133	320	76	19	1	0
cooked	1/2 cup	70	294	69	13	6	neg	Berries, strawberry	12 med	100	81	19	3	2	0
Soya beans, raw	1 tbsp	25	426	102	9	9	4	Cherries	20 med	100	201	48	12	1	0
canned	1/2 cup	100	466	111	11	10	4	Custard apple	1/2 med	75	230	55	12	1	0
Split peas, raw	1 tbsp	25	364	87	16	6	neg	Date, dried	5 whole	40	422	101	25	1	0
cooked	1/2 cup	90	433	103	19	7	neg	Fig, fresh	2 whole	95	161	30	8	1	0
STARCHY VEGETABLES *cooked edible portion*								Fig, dried	2 whole	30	272	65	16	1	0
Potato	1 med	120	330	70	16	3	0	Gooseberry, stewed, unsweetened	1/2 cup	125	78	19	4	1	0
Sweetcorn	1/2 cup	85	470	112	22	2	2	Grapefruit, fresh	half	120	133	32	6	1	0
Sweet potato	1/2 cup	120	377	92	21	2	0	Grapefruit, juice, unsweetened	1/2 cup	120	152	36	8	0	0
Yam	1/2 cup	120	473	113	27	3	0	Grapes	20	100	256	61	15	1	0
OTHER VEGETABLES								Honeydew melon	1/4 med	150	194	46	10	1	0
Where half a cup of cooked vegetables provides 5 grams or less of carbohydrate, we have classified them as 'low starch vegetables'. These vegetables are also low in kilojoules (calories), protein and fat, but high in vitamins, minerals and fibre. Include some in your meal plan every day.								Kiwifruit	1 med	60	124	29	6	1	0
								Lemon	1 med	50	48	12	2	0	0
								Lime	1 med	30	27	6	0	0	0

Kale, Kohlrabi, Lettuce, Marrow, Mushroom, Mung beans/sprouts, Onion, Parsley, Parsnip, Peas, Pumpkin, Radish, Silverbeet, Spinach, Summer squash, Swede, Tomato, Turnip, Watercress, Zucchini

*C = Carbohydrate   P = Protein   F = Fat   A = Alcohol   neg = negligible

Food Measure	Serve	g	Energy kJ	cal	C g	P g	F g
Lychee	8 whole	100	286	68	16	1	0
Mandarine	1 med	75	122	29	6	1	0
Mango	1 med	120	283	67	16	1	0
Nectarine	2 med	100	156	37	8	1	0
Orange	1 med	150	234	56	12	2	0
Orange, juice, commercial, unsweetened	1/2 cup	120	175	42	9	1	0
Passionfruit, pulp	1 med	20	39	9	1	1	0
Pawpaw	1 cup	240	296	70	16	0	0
Peach, fresh	1	110	145	35	7	1	0
Peach, canned, unsweetened	1 cup	220	230	55	13	2	0
Pear, fresh	1	150	317	76	19	0	0
Pear, canned, unsweetened	1 cup	200	220	53	13	0	0
Pineapple, fresh	1 slice	140	221	53	11	2	0
Pineapple, juice	1/2 cup	120	244	58	14	0	0
Pineapple, canned, unsweetened	2 slices	100	187	45	10	1	0
Plum	3	100	164	39	10	1	0
Prune, dried	6 med	50	343	82	20	1	0
Quince, stewed, unsweetened	1/2 cup	125	170	41	10	0	0
Raisin/sultana/currant	1 tbsp	13	136	33	8	0	0
Rhubarb, stewed, unsweetened	1/2 cup	130	33	8	1	1	0
Rock melon, Cantaloupe, small	half	200	182	43	10	2	0
Tamarillo, peeled	1 med	50	56	13	2	1	0
Watermelon	1 cup	220	211	50	11	1	0

*An average serve of many of the fruits in this list will contribute only a small amount of carbohydrate and kilojoules (calories). If the serve size (or part of a serve) contains 5 grams or less of carbohydrate, there is no need to count it as part of your meal plan. However, if you eat several serves of low-carbohydrate fruits throughout the day they will contribute significantly to your carbohydrate and kilojoule (calorie) intake.

MILK AND DAIRY PRODUCTS
Milk

Measure	Serve	g	kJ	cal	C	P	F
skim	250 mL	260	369	88	13	9	0
powder, skim	3 tbsp	33	499	119	17	12	0
evaporated, skim	1/2 cup	162	689	164	24	17	0
2% fat	250 mL	260	606	145	15	10	5
full cream	250 mL	260	707	169	12	9	10
powder, full cream	3 tbsp	27	554	132	11	7	7
evaporated, full cream	1/2 cup	162	1069	255	18	14	15

Cheese

Measure	Serve	g	kJ	cal	C	P	F
cottage, low-fat	1/2 cup	100	362	86	2	18	1
block, low-fat 7%		30	242	58	0	10	2
ricotta, low-fat		60	332	79	1	7	5
block, low-fat 18%		30	360	90	0	20	5
cheddar		30	504	120	0	8	10
cream		30	431	103	0	2	10

Yoghurt

Measure	Serve	g	kJ	cal	C	P	F
low-fat natural	1 small	200	420	110	0	13	12
full-cream, natural	1 small	200	650	155	13	9	8
diet yoghurt	1 small	200	380	90	13	9	0
low-fat flavoured/fruit	1 small	200	744	178	32	10	2
full-cream flavoured/fruit	1 small	200	826	197	32	10	4

Ice cream

Measure	Serve	g	kJ	cal	C	P	F
diet	2 level scoops	50 g	384	94	10	2	5

* There are many low-fat, and low-fat artificially sweetened ice creams available. Choose those with a fat content of less than 4.0 gms and less than 15 gms total CHO per 100 mL (2 level scoops).

PROTEIN FOODS
Meat and meat products

Food	Serve	g	kJ	cal	C	P	F
Beef, lean, minced		120	581	139	0	26	4
Beef, raw, lean only		120	602	144	0	26	4
Ham, leg, lean	1 slice	30	136	32	0	6	1
Lamb, raw, lean only		120	608	145	0	26	4
Liver		120	816	195	3	26	9
Luncheon meat	1 slice	30	321	77	1	4	6
Pork, raw, lean only		120	531	127	0	27	2
Pork sausage, cooked	2 thin	75	990	237	8	10	18
Salami, thin slices	3	30	538	128	0	7	11
Soya bean curd (tofu)	1/2 cup	110	303	72	2	8	6
Veal, raw, lean only		120	531	127	0	27	2

Poultry

Food	Serve	g	kJ	cal	C	P	F
Chicken, breast, no skin, raw		120	563	135	0	27	3

Fish and seafood

Food	Serve	g	kJ	cal	C	P	F
Fish, raw fillet	med	100	386	92	0	18	2
Oysters, raw	1/2 doz	60	130	31	0	6	1
Prawns, boiled		100	451	108	0	22	2
Tuna/salmon, canned in brine, drained	1/2 cup	90	411	98	0	20	2
Tuna, canned in oil, fish incl. oil	1/2 cup	90	1082	258	0	20	0

*C = Carbohydrate   P = Protein   F = Fat   A = Alcohol   neg = negligible

Eat & Enjoy   Food Lists

Food Measure	Serve	g	Energy kJ	cal	C g	P g	F g	Food	Serve mL	Energy kJ	cal	C g	A g
Eggs								*ALCOHOLIC BEVERAGES*					
Egg, hen, (55 g)	1 med	47	288	69	0	6	5	One standard drink = about 10 g alcohol and 335 kilojoules (80 calories) with the exception of alcohol-reduced drinks.					
Nuts								**Beer**					
Almonds, raw	1/3 cup	50	1168	278	2	5	27	Extra light beer, 1% alc.	200	135-210	32-50	8-10	2
Peanuts, raw	1/3 cup	50	1182	281	5	12	25	Light beer, 2-3% alcohol	200	190-250	46-60	4-6	4-6
Pecans, raw	1/3 cup	50	1379	328	11	4	33	Beer, 3.5-4% alcohol	200	335	80	6	7-8
Pinenuts, raw	2 tbsp	20	498	119	3	4	11	Diet ale, 3.5-4% alcohol	200	290	70	3	7-8
Peanut butter	1 tbsp	20	516	123	2	5	11	Stout	200	335	80	4	9
FATS								**Wine**					
Margarine, butter	1 tbsp	20	608	145	0	0	16	Wine, white, riesling	100	350	85	neg	12
Oil, blended, polyunsaturated	1 tbsp		702	168	0	0	19	Wine, red, claret	100	350	85	neg	12
Cream, thickened	2 tbsp	40	547	131	1	1	14	Champagne, dry	100	350	65	neg-2	12
Dressing, French, commercial	2 tbsp	40	625	149	3	0	16	Wine, white sauternes	100	370	90	4	11
Mayonnaise, light, commercial	1 tbsp	20	258	62	3	0	5	**Other**					
								Spirits, brandy, gin, whisky, rum	30	276	66	0	10
Olives, in brine	4 med	27	113	27	0	0	3	Sherry, dry	60	335	80	1	9
Potato chips/fries	10 chips	85	394	94	2	15	2	Vermouth, dry	60	335	80	1	11
Potato crisps, plain, small packet	1	25	526	126	12	2	8	Cider	200	335	80	2	10
								Sherry, sweet	60	365	90	4	11
Popcorn, plain		20	353	84	14	3	2	Vermouth, sweet	60	365	90	4	11
								Liqueurs	20	300	70	6	7
								Port	60	260	60	8	10

*C = Carbohydrate P = Protein F = Fat A = Alcohol neg = negligible

INDEX

Acesulfame-K 25
Adolescents 47-9
After-dinner treats
  date rolls 197
  frozen fruit 198
  fruit cheese 197
  rum balls 198
Alcohol 23
Appetisers and snacks
  accompaniment for dips 61
  asparagus rolls 61
  cheese puffs 66
  chick pea savoury 66
  chicken liver paté 63
  chicken spread 69
  Chinese dumplings 69
  dolmades 65
  moong dhal 64
  mushroom starter 68
  pumpernickel savouries 61
  vegetable samosas 67
  wholemeal salmon slices 68
Artificial sweeteners 20, 25-7
Aspartame 25, 27
Australian Dietary
  Guidelines 16

Baking
  apple and apricot slice 195
  apple-nut streusel
    wholemeal cake 196
  bread, wholemeal 191
  carrot cake 192
  cookies, Chris's 189
  damper, wholemeal 188
  fruit (Christmas) cake 194
  loaf, date and walnut 196
  mince tarts 194-5
  muffins, banana 189
  muffins, bluestone 193
  muffins, herby corn 188
  pastry, wholemeal 190
  pikelets 190-1
  scones 192-3
  scones, fruit 193
Biscuits
  accompaniment for dip 61
Blood fat levels, high 46

Blood glucose level *8-9*, 11,
  12, 13, 18, 20, 32, 42, 43
  impact of exercise 51-2, 53
  normal 10
Blood pressure, high 45
Bread
  accompaniment for dip 61
Breakfasts 57
  coddled egg 59
  liquid breakfast 58
  Meg's muesli 58

Calories (kilojoules)
  artifical sweeteners 26
  energy source 15
  products low in 27
Carbohydrates 14
  daily serves 32-3
  foods 8, 16-18, 22
  modified products 27
  needs 32-3, 53
Cereals 17
  better choices 30
Cheese 22
Chicken
  apricot 113
  Caesar's 110
  Chinese, with sweetcorn
    soup 72
  enchiladas 116
  five-spice 111
  green pea, spinach and
    chicken soup 71
  liver paté 63
  mustard seed sauce 111
  risotto, golden 115
  saté 114-15
  soy 117
  spread 69
  stock 71
  strawberry and peppercorn
    sauce 112-13
  tikka 114
Children 47-9
Cholesterol 46
Conserves
  dried apricot 60
  fresh strawberry 59

Cracked wheat 145
Crêpes 82. *see also* Pancakes
  flambéed 179
  savoury fillings 83-4
  Suzette 178
Curry
  paste 164
  powder 164
Curry accompaniments
  banana-yoghurt relish 102
  cucumber and yoghurt 102
  tomato and mint salad 102
Custard. *see* Sauces, sweet
Cyclamate 25-6, 27

Dairy products 22, 50
Date and fig spread 60
Desserts
  apple layer cake 167
  baked apples with orange
    and strawberry sauce
    176-7
  baked custard 178
  baked yoghurt slice 182
  berry salad (mixed) and
    lemon cream 174
  cheesecake, lemon and
    cinnamon 187
  crêpes 178-9
  dumplings, old-fashioned
    176
  fruit compote, English 177
  fruit crumble 172
  fruit flummery, golden 182-3
  fruit strudel 168
  ginger pears 175
  ice-cream, crunchy peach
    186
  lemon delicious 169
  mousse, mocha 183
  oranges, spiced 170
  pancakes 178-80
  pineapple, hot Jamaican
    174
  pudding, bread and butter
    54, 184
  pudding, Christmas 185

pudding, fruity baked rice 175
pudding, Queen's 184-5
pudding, summer 172-3
pumpkin pie 173
rice, creamy 170
ricotta raisin 169
rock melon sorbet with blackcurrant or raspberry sauce 181
strudel, apple 168
strudel, apricot 168
strudel, banana 168
sweet potato and pecan pie 171
Diabetes
  definition 8-10
  diet 12, 13
  exercise 13
  gestational 47
  insulin-dependant 10, 52
  management 12-24
  mellitus 10-11
  non-insulin dependent 10, 11, 51
  products 27
  rules 12-13
  statistics 6
  symptoms 9-10
  tablets 11, 39, 44
  Type 1 10
  Type 2 10, 11
  uncontrolled 11
Diabetes Australia 7
Diarrhoea 44
Dietitians 6
Dressings
  curry 161
  herbed tomato 161
  Italian 160
  orange, creamy 161
  orange and soy 160
  yoghurt, creamy 160
Drinks
  50/50 swirl 199
  apricot cooler 199
  cherries and leben 200
  hot claret punch 200
  hot milk sleeper 200
  Irish coffee 199

Kiwi cooler 200
orange buttermilk 199
sangria 200
strawberry granita 199

Eating out 40
Eggs 21
Energy needs 31
Entrees and light meals
  beef and bean burritos (wholemeal) 79
  Bombay burgers with cucumber and yoghurt sauce 81
  crêpes and pancakes 82-3
  crêpes and pancakes, savoury fillings for 83-4
  filo rolls 85-6
  gado gado 86
  harlequin noodle salad 80
  pasties 85
  prosciutto and rock melon (cantaloupe) 80
  spinach ravioli with fresh tomato sauce 81
Ethnic restaurants 40
Exercise 13
  adjusting food intake 53
  blood glucose level 51-2, 53
  fluids 53
  hypoglycaemia 52-3
  ready reckoner for carbohydrate intake 53

Fats 14, 18
  foods with 20-1
  needs 32, 56
  saturated vegetable 46
Fibre 15, 18, 33, 57
  foods with 19
Fillings
  potato. see Potatoes
  sandwich 62
  savoury, for crêpes and pancakes 83-4
Filo rolls 85-6
Fish and seafood 21
  cooking methods 87-8
  crab and zucchini quiche 92
  curried tuna and rice casserole 88

fish in orange sauce 89
mussels a la grecque 94
paella 93
pasta and smoked trout 92
piquant fish in foil 89
salmon mornay 94
sauces for 88
seafood canneloni 95
seafood pasta 90
vegetable-stuffed trout 91
whole fish in ginger 90-1
Flavour 56
Food
  carbohydrate modified 27
  energy source 15
  guidelines to choosing 16-22
  labels 28-9
  low calorie 27
  nutrient composition 29
  processed 18
  sugar free 28
  value list 201-4
Fructose 26
Fruit 17
  accompaniment for dips 61

Gestational diabetes 47
Glucose 8, 9, 10
Glycaemic index 18
Glycosuria 9

Hyperglycaemia 11, 42-3, 53
Hypoglycaemia
  prevention 43, 52
  symptoms 42
  treatment 44
  what to do 42-3
  why it happens 43

Ice-cream 186
Illness
  diarrhoea 44
  food intake during 44
  vomiting 44
Insulin 9, 24, 39, 44
  exercise 51
  injections 39
  sport 51
  timing meals 39
  types 39

Insulin-Dependent Diabetes Mellitus (IDDM) 10, 52
Islets of Langerhans 10

Ketosis 10
Kilojoules. *see* Calories

Lactose 26
Lamb. *see* Meat
Liver, Balinese spiced 112

Mannitol 26
Marinades
  red wine zap 162
  Singapore sizzler 162
  spicy lamb 162
Meals
  plans 31, 33, 34
  plans, samples of 35-8
  timing 39
Meat 21. *see also* Chicken; Poultry
  beef, pickled 104
  beef curry 101
  chilli con carne 104-5
  fillet, baked with cherry sauce 106
  lamb, Indian, in spinach sauce 107
  lamb, Mogul 108
  lamb, skewered 102
  lamb with garlic and mustard 106
  liver, Balinese spiced 112
  Malaysian fried rice noodles 98
  meat a la pizzaiola 103
  meatballs in tomato sauce 100
  meatloaf with spicy barbecue sauce 99
  pork, Chinese stir-fry 97
  pork tango 96
  rabbit, sweet and sour with prunes 119
  rabbit casserole 118
  steak and black bean sauce 105
  veal mango 109
Meatless dishes
  bean bake, jumping 120

bubble and squeak 130
cheese and spinach rolls 123
curry, vegetable 125
fettuccine, spinach 129
gnocchi, potato 126-7
gnocchi, semolina with tomato and basil sauce 126
lasagne, vegetarian 122
omelette, Spanish 124-5
pie, Mexicale with cornmeal dumplings 128
pie, Tibetan 124
pita pizza 127
quiche, claytons 130
vegetable loaf 121
Menus 33, 40
Milk products 22, 50
Minerals 15
Mixers. *see* Soft drinks
Modifying recipes 54-5
Monosodium glutamate (MSG) 45

Nocturia 9
Non-insulin Dependent Diabetes Mellitus (NIDDM) 10, 11, 51
Nutrition
  information on 29, 201-4
  principles 13-15
Nuts 22

Oral hypoglycaemic agents. *see* Diabetes tablets

Pancakes
  apple and sultana 179
  berry and cheese 179
  buckwheat with blueberry sauce 180
  flambéed 179
  savoury fillings 83-4
Pancreas 9, 10, 11
Pasties 85
Pastry. *see* Baking
Pickles
  mango, fresh 163
  tomato relish 162
Polydipsia 9

Polyuria 9
Pork. *see* Meat
Portions 32
Potatoes
  curried with cauliflower 138
  curry with eggplant and pea 136
  diced, parsleyed 132
  duchess 135
  fillings 134
  gnocchi 126-7
  jacket 134
  scalloped 133
  sweet, patties 137
Poultry 21. *see also* Chicken
Pregnancy 47
Protein 14
  foods 21-2, 50
  needs 32
Pudding. *see* Desserts
Pulses 17, 22

Quiche
  claytons 130
  crab and zucchini 92

Rabbit. *see* Meat
Recipes, modifying. *see* Modifying recipes
Relish, tomato 162
Rice
  creamy 170
  crunchy peasant 143
  curried carrot soup 76
  curried tuna casserole 88
  fruity baked pudding 175
  mushroom and pecan 137
  salad, crunchy 153
  spiced with peas 140
Roughage. *see* Fibre

Saccharin 26, 27
Salads
  asparagus and green bean 146
  avocado, spinach and tofu 146
  broad bean and smoked salmon 151
  broccoli, beanshoots and snowpeas with lemon 147

coleslaw 151
curried pasta 148
curried sweet potato and banana 150
fettucine salmon 152
fruity noodle 147
ginger carrots 146
harlequin noodle mushroom 146
orange and cucumber 146
potato, new 149
potato, tangy 150
riata 152
rice, crunchy 153
spinach Valentino 148
tabbouleh 149
tomato and onion 146
tossed 153
Salt 45, 56
  substitutes 45
Sandwich fillings 62
Sauces, savoury
  black bean 157
  champagne, green 159
  cheese 155
  cherry 154
  cucumber and yoghurt 158
  plum 163
  ratatouille 157
  saté (peanut) 155
  strawberry and peppercorn 158
  sweet and sour 159
  tomato and basil 156
  vegetable, fresh 156
  white 154
Sauces, sweet
  blueberry 165
  brandy 166
  custard 166
  custard, orange 166
  topping, creamy whip 165
Seafood. see Fish and seafood
Seasonings
  curry paste 164
  curry powder 164
Seeds 22
Serves 32-3, 201
Shift work 41
Side dishes, vegetable 131
Snacking 33

Soft drinks 23
Sorbitol 26
Soups
  beef and bean 77
  broccoli and sweetcorn 75
  chicken stock 71
  Chinese chicken and sweetcorn 72
  corn chowder 72
  curried carrot and rice 76
  gazpacho 78
  green pea, spinach and chicken 71
  hot and sour 73
  Hungarian 75
  minestrone 70
  orange borscht 78
  pork and vegetable noodle 76
  Singapore noodle 74
  souper douper pumpkin 77
Soya milk 51
Sport. see Exercise
Starches 18
Sucralose 26
Sugar 19-20, 56
  products free of 28
  refined 17
Sweeteners. see Artificial sweeteners

Takeaway meals 41
Travel 41
Triglycerides 46

Veal. see Meat
Vegans 51
Vegetables 17. see also Meatless dishes
  accompaniment for dips 61
  beets, hot shredded 144
  broccoli, lemon 131
  brussel sprouts, curried with almonds 135
  cabbage, red, sweet and sour 143
  curried potatoes and cauliflower 138
  curry, potato, eggplant and pea 136
  eggplant Neapolitan 141

  Julienne 144
  leek and apple 132
  lettuce, braised 131
  mushroom and pecan rice 137
  mushroom stroganoff 138
  onions, braised 131
  parsnips, orange-glazed 142
  potato, sweet, patties 137
  potatoes, diced parsleyed 132
  potatoes, duchess 135
  potatoes, jacket 134
  potatoes, scalloped 133
  pumpkin and mushrooms 132
  pumpkin pie 173
  rice, crunchy peasant 143
  rice, spiced with peas 140
  side dishes 131
  snow peas and asparagus 132
  spinach and spring onions 131
  stir-fried 145
  succotash 132
  vegeballs 142
  vegetables en brochette 141
  zucchini and carrot rings 132
  zucchini and tomato bake 139
  zucchini Creole 133
Vegetarians 49-51
  daily intake for lacto-ovo 50
  food guidelines 49-50
Vitamins
  fat-soluble 14
  water-soluble 14
Vomiting 44

Water 15
Weight control 13, 24
Wheat, cracked 145

Yoghurt 22

Zucchini. see Vegetables